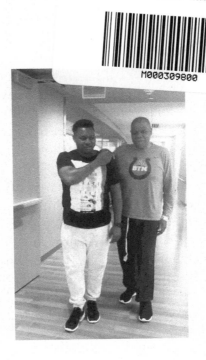

INTRODUCTION BY
JOHN SCHOGER

Standing at six feet, five inches tall, James Thornton has always been a mountain of a man. With an infectious smile and a laugh that fills the room as much as his physical presence, James is a larger-than-life character.

I first met James at a Bible study my wife and I attended at the home of Matt and Claire Hamilton in Columbus in 2017. It was a perfect summer evening and James could not be missed - jovial, well dressed, and standing a head above all the other guests. Meeting James for the first time, I received his welcoming hand, a broad smile and his complete attention.

That evening was one day after James' birthday and following the study, his girlfriend Lisa Showe (now his beautiful wife) surprised James with a cake and we all sang happy birthday. The giant was brought to tears. He thanked everyone and said that he had never felt so welcomed in his life.

In the coming months I would get to know James through Core Community, a weekly men's fellowship and bible study. James was regularly attending, growing in the Word and always had much to share. Engaging and charismatic, I - along with everyone else - cherished his friendship.

But on June 6, 2018, James's life held in the balance. Worried after not hearing from James, an alert was sounded by his friend, Deborah Johnson who was to meet with him that morning. By afternoon, friends Reggie Moore and Leon Lewis went to his apartment building searching where they found him unconscious. He had suffered a Stroke and lay unresponsive for up to 20 hours.

Rushed to Riverside Hospital, the prognosis for James was grim. It was doubtful that he would live. And, if by some miracle he survived, chances are that he would never walk or regain the ability to speak.

James Thornton, the public speaker who had successfully navigated a professional career with the National Football League, USA Track & Field, and global banking giant UBS, was silent. The college football player who overcame childhood poverty and hardship to travel the globe for broadcasting networks and the U.S. Olympic Committee was grounded.

But God had a plan for James. Able to hear but not speak, James focused on God's Word and became a listener of others. Forced to slow down, he gained patience. One syllable at a time, he regained his speech. And one step at a time, he strengthened his gait.

God was using the Stroke to change the mountain of a man *into* a mountain. Set in place and time, one cannot help to be drawn to a mountain. A mountain forces you to look up to the heavens and glorify God. In the same way, James' story, his heart and his character draws everyone to him, but he directs all the glory up to the Father and Creator.

As all great mountains birth streams, James now refreshes others through his writings and encouragement, what he fondly calls, *dripping*. Providing hope to Stroke survivors and their loved ones, and raising the awareness and prevention of Strokes, James takes the love and grace he receives daily from God and redistributes it to others.

James is an inspiration to me and I am proud to call him my friend and brother in Christ. I cannot thank him enough for teaching me to slow down, to listen to the Lord and for allowing me to join him on this fabulous journey.

To the readers of this book, the pages that follow are in James' own, genuine voice, post-stroke. They capture his miraculous journey from near death silence and having to relearn to speak and write, to being an inspiring author. Unedited and in his authentic style, enjoy James' short stories with the same Grace and Mercy that he affords others. Most of all, enjoy reading this book because James feels so great to be able to communicate his love and gratitude with you through writing again.

John Schoger

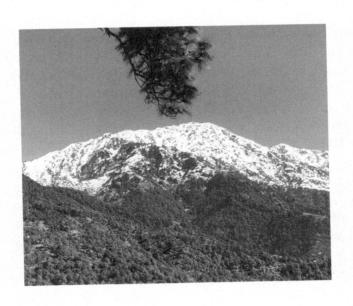

KEY LESSON TO LEARN...
TOGETHER

When people have a Stroke they cannot speak at first. Maybe they were a "great speaker" before or talk in a "soft voice". But no matter what they were before...now they are "listeners" again. Like a "child being guided through life" for the very first time. Starting on Day 1 those around them are constantly talking because as family or caregivers you care. But the familiar voice that you need to hear from us is gone. The sounds or grunts we make you do not recognize. So you do what naturally comes next...making plans and decisions on our behalf as best as you can. We both are in "uncharted territory" for sure and it is why we need each other. But it takes you making the "first step" before I walk out the door of a hospital. Then on to the "next step". Both of us have the rehabilitation of our minds and body. But it starts with "Step 1" that we both need to focus on. You slow your mind down to a pedestrian pace which may be painful at the start. But once it happens it gets easier to do in time. We need all your love shown as best possible shown to us. As a Stroke Survivor to know you are out there "talking back to us" by reading to us. Nothing else matters at that point because all control of everything has been lost. Given up the tragic circumstances that we are now in...together. But with a "teamwork approach" you will be able to figure things out..."one step" at a time. You see adversity introduces us all to ourselves again. We all are a "Survivor" of something. So "teamwork" in all facets of this game is needed to get through this "uncertain time". While it does take a lot of "work and perseverance" the benefits can be life changing. The biggest one is you have the freedom to "make a choice" to help another...it is not easy to do. But you did. So when you look at this picture you will want to "focus on the mountain" but instead cast your gaze on "the tree". That is our first and best step...together. Because no one is in "control of this situation"...neither you nor me. This is my premise for writing and sharing this book to the world.

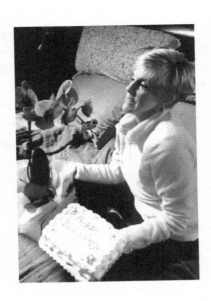

FOREWORD

"James you have brought WARMTH" by Mrs. Lisa Showe my Wife. We were married on November 16, 2019. My Stroke occurred overnight June 5, 2018 and I was found the next day in the afternoon.

"WHERE there has been cold, you have brought warmth; where there was darkness, you have brought light." Our miracle lies in the path we have chosen together. I enter this marriage with you knowing that the true magic is not to avoid change but to follow the path together, hand in hand. Let us commit to the miracle of making each day work together.

Whatever lies ahead, good or bad, we will face together. Distance may test us for a time and time may try us, but if we look to each other first we will always see a friend. I believe in you, the person you will grow to be and the couple we will be together. With all my heart I take you James as my husband, acknowledging your faults and strengths as you do mine.

You have been my best friend, mentor, playmate, confident and my greatest challenge. But most importantly you are the love of my life and you make me happier than I could ever imagine and more loved than I thought possible.

You have made me a better person, as our love for each other is reflected in the way I live my life. So I am truly blessed to be a part of your life which as of today becomes our life together.

What can I say that I haven't already said? What can I provide you that I haven't already given? My body, my mind, my soul and my heart. They are all yours.

Everything that I am and everything that I have belonged to you long before today. And I promise that it shall all be yours forever. I will be yours forever. I will follow you anywhere you go and anywhere you lead me..."HAND IN HAND".

Love is a short word, easy to spell and difficult to define and impossible to live without. LOVE is work, but most of all love is realizing that every hour every minute every second of it was worth it because we did it together. On this special day James I give to you, in the presence of God and all these family and friends my promise to be faithful and supportive and to always make our family's love and happiness my priority. I will be yours in plenty and in want, in sickness and in health in failure and in triumph. I will dream with you, celebrate with you and walk beside you through whatever our lives may bring. You are my person, my LOVE and my LIFE today and always."

International Business

James Thornton has spent the majority of his career building a highly successful portfolio of international and US-based ventures in the areas of sports and business development. As a "global citizen" he continues to amass a world-class rolodex and nurtures a network of significant relationships in the United Kingdom, Germany, Spain, Netherlands and other EU countries, as well as in China, Australia, and Brazil.

James uses experience to forge unique business partnerships by creating customized networking roadmaps to generate client introductions that yield mutually beneficial results. By taking a collaborative approach the firm's value proposition is achieved. "Use acquired knowledge, a broad network of influential contacts with market intelligence to provide "Access & Introductions" for the client that builds a strategic alliance and optimal returns."

In 2005, UBS hired Mr. Thornton to design and lead the firm's first-ever minority business unit to manage relationships with high growth suppliers, minority businesses and affinity groups globally. As Executive Director of the Business & Diversity Partnerships Group, the unique operating model focused on both supplier diversity and diverse sector business development. Applying his strategic thinking skills which included the involvement of the Americas and EMEA Regions Employee Network Groups, he introduced UBS banking teams to Native American and First Nations (Canada) tribal contacts, minority business owners and entrepreneurs around the world. Accomplishments were - an increased brand identity within the sector and $1.7 billion in new banking business from 2007-2012 to the Investment Bank, Wealth Management and Global Asset Management divisions.

Prior to joining UBS, his prior roles included working with the National Football League (in London and New York), USA Track & Field, the US Olympic Committee, production member of various US TV networks, and consultant for five Summer Olympic Games, including London 2012 and one Winter Olympic Game in Sotchi. As was a spokesperson for "The H.O.P.E. Program" a health & wellness initiative for former NFL Players sponsored by Covidien and NFL Players Association at the time.

"REINTRODUCING MYSELF"...TO ME AGAIN BY JAMES THORNTON

Thank you for taking this "Journey" with me. The brain is a mystery. When you wake up from a coma and have no "memories"...all you can do is wink. "Once" for yes. "Two" for no. Its Alzheimers...yet in reverse. It does not matter your culture or religion when you cannot speak. For once it is "just silence" you live in. So these stories will tell you two important things. The first 4 Chapters represent my "Attention Span" these days. The 5th Chapter represents my fingers and how I learn to "count again". This new life of having a Stroke teaches me daily "its not being brave until I am afraid" as I learned what concrete and grass feels like when I fall on them...again. Learning from a different lense now what I thought was "true or false" is really..."gray". Prejudice knows no reason yet my mind have been both "my Defense and Prosecutor attorneys". Having never been inside a jail cell literally...in my mind I am "lock up" seeking freedom yet "sentence was commuted" the day of the Stroke. Where all I had done in life disappeared because my mind was erased. So now this verse resonates..."The thief's purpose is to steal and kill and destroy. My purpose is to give them a rich and satisfying life". It is from John 10:10 NLT. For me Bible verses do matter if I can see them in action versus preaching to me. For I am an "infant in growns up body" taking a village to help raise me again in this "new world". Having "faith in you" was something you had to earn back then. Yet "He" saved my life while I slept on my bedroom floor as I watched from...a close distance. Deciding to send me back to this world when no medical intervention would save my life that day.

My ex-girlfriend became my wife when she did not have to and is "head of the village" I reside in. I used to do more before this Stroke. Yet I am still "Mr James Thornton" just "reclaim now". This "redemption" was paid in full a long time ago but I could not see it then. Today my "imperfections and success" are on full display...for all to see. Me standing in front of you today is a "miracle" so focus on "my messages" and not the text. Editing with "your heart and mind" versus a pen. Reading my words with love and humility allows them to "breathe" in your soul. Use your "access" into my world of surviving a Stroke to see that fate can be cruel...if we allow it. Whether a family member or caregivers or a just friend we are all "Survivors". So lets not focus on our circumstance but rejoice about the "Life" we have today. Taking one step at a time in this "sea of information overload" we swim in daily. But you can find your "North Star" also. It is your hands...just grasp it tightly and hold on. You see...delays in life do not mean you are "denied" so defy logic and listen to your heart.

"REINTRODUCING MYSELF"...TO ME AGAIN
BY JAMES THORNTON

As Stroke Survivors we have "retrain the Brain" in the following areas:

- we are "mute" in the beginning of the illness.

- we can hear you from Day 1 but no one can hear "us".

- we have an attention span of between 0-30 minutes as the start building back up slowly over time.

- we have various forms of "asphisa" which means we learn everything over again from speaking to spelling and learning how to write...again.

- we try to regain all of our mental and cognitive capabilities.

- we have to remember what to do with all of our bodily functions also.

For me in addition:

- I talk with a "stutter now" but it is better than being "silenced by others".

- my "ability to assume" has completely disappeared as a result of this Stroke so I ask questions now without judgement.

- my mind focuses on "one step... one door" at a time completing the task as best as I can before moving on.

As a result of a Stroke we are still experiencing all the same things you do...just in different ways now. "Wins" are great to celebrate. Raising an arm or a foot higher than yesterday and learning how to speak and write...all are awesome. These "small things" that most consider routine is what I helped others to attain now. On days when I am "struggling"...I just have to think about somewhere out there is someone worse off than me. You have a choice to make daily...to "Survive" or "Thrive". So welcome to my "New World". ☀

Chapter 1

THE BEGINNING -
"ONCE A MAN TWICE A CHILD..."
-EDITH "MAMAE" D. WEST
POINT GA "MY 2ND MOM"
AND COUSIN

Strokes Explained "By The Numbers"

Who: *Strokes do not discriminate. They affect all ages and demographics.*

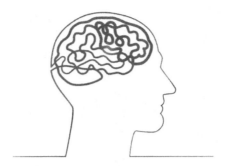

BY JAMES THORNTON A.K.A. "STROKE OF GENIUS"

You know having this Stroke has been interesting. Being mute to being able to speak has been interesting. Asking people questions to remember things they tell me has been interesting. When you have a Stroke you lose part of your memory in some cases. For me this happen. I regained my voice yet still needed to ask questions to people. Now it is a characteristic of my being. My friend Alison who suffered a Stroke is the same way. We ask questions to get clarity for information in order to engage the person thoughtfully. So why does not everybody ask questions first of each other...it would eliminate a lot of confusion. More importantly it would give us answers "straight from the horses mouth". I know for sure it will give us a better understanding of each other. We assume and speculate so much in this world. Maybe you too need a..Stroke of Genius.

HEAVEN

I do not know why but last night it was placed on my mind to share what heaven was like for me. I was in a pitch black room when this came to me even though the actual room I was in the floor lamp was on. So here goes my story... I had life-saving experience that happen and honestly drew me closer to God. First I feel no pain or discomfort during this time. What I did experience was a JOY that has not been matched since. It was like the day I signed my papers to attend college on a football scholarship. But I was on "Gods team"... with the joy and sacrifices made along with pride of how I was going to serve him now. I had made it to the big league. I was ready to take my place alongside him and do the work required of me. NO check that..."offered to me". I did not see angels or other things while in his presence...just God speaking as I listen. As I quickly arrived there I was back on this earth waking up in the hospital. This is my story. But that glimpse told me everything I need to know. God loves me. He wants me to treat my neighbor as myself...and make myself available to be use anyway he sees fit.

6 QUESTIONS I HAD

1. Is there a God? 🙏
2. What is Life? ☆
3. Who is God? 🌈
4. Why did God create me? 👥
5. Who am I? 👁
6. What do I do? 👤

As we explore ourselves to find out these things he will reveal himself to us. In his time though not ours. I have been trying to answer these questions for about 3 years. So before my Stroke. I would get close to an answer to one and it felt great. But trying to answer them all at the same time I could not. So I would start over...and over...and over. Now post-stroke I am still answering these questions. But here is the difference now. I just live out my answer to them all...its "Love". "Love for God". "Love" for myself. "Love" for other people. Keep learning a little more about myself each day...it is on the table too. Do your very best in life each day. That is all that we can ask of ourselves. And grow yourself. Start with small things and soon they will grow into much bigger things. Do this and you will be well on your way. But "listening" first...then engaging with the person. And then just ask God to reveal it to you too. But it starts with YOU and no one else.

HOT 3 MONTHS...

My Stroke happened over a summer...after surviving to be sent back I was visiting a "hot desert" for the first 3 months. Here is the deal about the ordeal. My teacher was in "Teaching mode" all the time. And he never disappointed and failed me. So this is what I learned on this part of my "Journey Back"...

1. I was functioning "mute" first of all...seriously I could not speak for 2 of those 3 months. Then the "Silence" was replaced with what I describe as gibberish.

2. And when you cannot talk everybody wants to chat with you.

3. And they talked about everything so let your imagination run wild.

4. Yet I listened because I had no choice. Gods "teaching moment" had arrived to show me I was not and would not be able to control anything under "his Watch" of the sun and moon.

But it did not stop there with these lessons. I am still learning today:

1. Everyone wants to be heard.

2. It's tough to talk when people are trying to speak "over"..."through"...and "around" each other.

3. We need to "think and reflect" before anything else happens.

4. I LISTEN first and am SLOW to speak... if it all.

5. Show you the "3 forms of Love" that he showed me that fateful day.

No pressure from me in any way because I want to "help you...help yourself". But "How...What...Why and Where" you may ask. I would too. Back in the day of old I leaned on my "own understanding and knowledge" about such things also. Yet now things have become much simpler and plain to me...

"How"- He gave me back what he originally took away.

"What" - My life...yet it operates "His way now".

"Why" - He is coming back and by showing you through my "imperfections" he can still use me now to help you...in my "NEW LIFE".

"Where" - When "you need it"...not when I want you to have. It is a "fluid" situation between us. So now you know about my transformation. And "how I live" in the principles of Philippians 1:20-28. Read this first...then digest at your own pace. Only then will you know "my story" and then we can talk about yours.

THE JOURNEY BACK

I am watching on movie and this scene the pilot of the craft is all ALONE in his spaceship. He was sent up ALONE...as the Cosmonaut. Theres no one to talk to up there...it was the very first time. He only had "his thoughts" to keep him occupied. For the first 3 months I could not speak a word to just uttering complete gibberish to those listening. They told me I had the "Mother Of All Strokes" laying on my bedroom floor for 20+

hours before being found. And once found the doctors said it would be a "true miracle" if I woke up out of the coma. For they had done all they could...which was nothing because I had past their "time limit" by a lot of hours. So there I lay in Gods hands. There is no one else to talk...but him. But like that Cosmonaut in my mind I was "thinking" about what had occurred. Answering questions...all them. If you ever had a Stroke this all sounds familiar to you. Your mind is clear and you are "speaking on your head" but no one can hear. So this is where "we" decide..."give up or fight like hell". Because to our loved ones and friends they can see only what in front of them. We are talking in our minds yet they "cannot read our mind". They want us to talk and speak to them again. To let them know how we are feeling. We are SPEAKING yet they cannot HEAR US. Paying attention with "an impaired mind" takes patience from "me and you". You want information from me but in "your time" not mine. So you give up. I want to focusing on the one thing important to me...saving my life. Post-stroke my focus has been narrowed down to a single thing. All my "sensory information" is jumbled like a jigsaw puzzle. Pieces are there and just need to be put back together...again. My abilities to track things whether "in space" or "inside my head" have changed forever. From that hospital bed through to all the rehabilitation required..."I am trying". But what comes back...will "ultimately come back in its own time". You are rushing around in a hurry...yet as a "Stroke Survivor" it is not a good match. That "hurried world of the rat race" does not help or interest me now. All because I was given something back more important...LIFE. You see we all are disabled. So my takeaway from this experience...it is not about me anymore. Sharing my stories to help others to see what is inside of me and them...is "the same". My life now is enjoying watching others "blossoms into the beautiful flower that they are". It is this "Inner Beauty" we all should seek in each other. I have been given a second chance...I relish in this "beautiful side" of life. Because the "barrier of loneliness" has been replaced. It is you and me now sharing LOVE for each other...in my "new world".

BLESSING FROM DIFFICULTIES

I carried grudges against others. I retaliated when judged by others. I used to get really upset with people no matter what. I would let anger boil up inside of me until it erupted. I did coveted things others had. I "control" my actions therefore...I "control my life". Then something happened. Those feelings and subsequent actions left my life. God transformed me. Now I know my weakness is…"his strength". I know that he loves me...even when I did not love myself. He wants me to practice using the "grace and mercy" he shows me...to others. For now I am truly weak. Vulnerable to him. Seeking him out. And now with him I can take on this world with a different perspective. I live to help people figure out what they are seeking - Career Wise...Personally...or Spiritually. Yet it means meeting them where they are now in their life. Not where I want them to be.

ASSUMPTION

"Why is it so hard being friends with a Jew." one man asked another. "Try being one." was the response of the other man. - from a Play

This is what I know…"until we ask we do not know". That goes for anything in life. All I know if I do not ask a question yet come up with my own answer...that is "an assumption". Therefore my "assumption" will lead my thoughts on that topic. When in reality I just need to ask the question. But in doing so we must be prepared to get an answer that goes against what we believe in. And that rubs us as people the wrong way at times. Yet for me I think it offers a chance to converse on topics. While understanding that we might "agree to disagree" at the end there is a "conversation". I thought this exchange between these two guys was interesting. What I learned from this exchange is…"there are always two sides to every story". Yet when we do not want to hear it…to understand the other side we are short changing ourselves. Because we all should be able to learn until the day we die. Then again we have a choice to decide to make in that case. So make the right choice. I believe you will.

LOSING CONCENTRATION

Losing concentration will kill you as a football player. It causes you to make mistakes that you do not make normally. It causes you to "press down" on the next play…if you have another down. It causes you to play with unsettling caution on the next play also. Players will tell you that they do not think about it….their lying. Its normal. It happens. What saves the player is when they "stash it away mentally". Believing in a higher power is the same thing. Believe in something we cannot see or touch is a true belief. When we lose concentration as Christians…we have forgotten how we came to God. For me it was a long road…filled with "alternative lanes". But HE still loved me. So much that now "HE" helps me not lose concentration. When it does happens I just "re-focus" by trying to help others. It does happen for sure. Like a football player we have to "recognize" it first…then get back on "our horse".

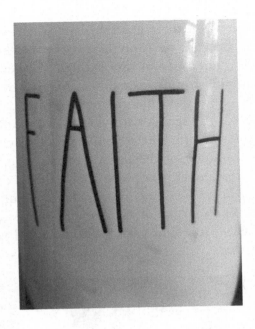

LEARNING IS TOUGH

What does this mean if you do not know about God or you are unsure if "he is even there" in your life. You see...I know all about this subject from firsthand experiences. There were times in my life I knew there was a God...but he did not live in "my zip code". So armed with what I knew back then...I had both "successes and failures" in my life. Living "my life" the only way I knew how. In "my way" or "you could hit the highway". It was my "terms and conditions" only. But then the Stroke came...and changed everything forever. It took away..."all of my memories". It took away..."my ability to talk". It took away..."my chance write again". I was left inside my head "talking away" but no one else could hear me..."on the outside". As I struggled each day..."to find myself". I found out what was always there. It was..."God". To help him make Disciples from "all nations". Does not matter to me your "color...cash...or culture". By using "my circumstances now"...he show you there a better way to tackle this thing called "life". Because we "only know what we know". And sometimes it is not a lot...or "not enough". So never focus on "where you come from". Focus on..."where you are now". With a little effort and time on your part...you can help us "Disciples too". You see they still come "1 at a time" to God. That take time and much help from others. But you could be the "planter...waterer or the cultivator" for sure. That is all you need to remember. I know this for a fact because I have been where you are. Walking in your shoes..."but to where". This picture represents all of us...from all our "walks of life". And guess what...I would never have thought I would have said "Yes" either.

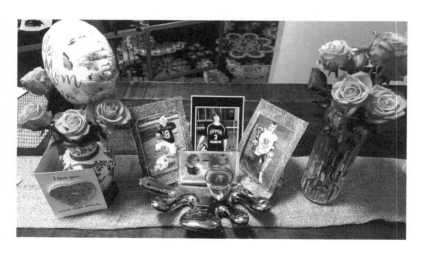

RESPECT…

> "She is clothed with strength and dignity, and she laughs
> without fear of the future. She carefully watches every-
> thing in her household and suffers nothing from laziness.
> Her children stand and bless her. Her husband praises her"
> —Proverbs 31:25, 27-28 NLT

I listened to a song that says what we all want in life…"Respect"
by ADEVA. Before you turn your nose up at me listen to it.
Its how we should treat each other. I got married for the first
time and it will be my only time. And that means there are
going to be times when we wont agree. Because that is life.
Yet I have give her this "Respect" that ADEVA sings about.
More importantly we need to support and encourage one
another constantly. Even when it is painful to do because of
how I am feeling. These "Anthem of words" are true and spot
on. We have to get out of our own way. I have to depend on
"God" now to help when I cannot help myself. She deserves
my "Respect" daily. So do not take home any problems from
other situations occurring during your day - relationships…
work…etc. For our time together is "reserved". Just like we
want "Respect" daily…we must also give it "Respect".

OPTIMISTIC

I am writing today sharing this thought…being "Optimistic"
in this life of ours. You see if we do not have it we can only
blame ourselves…me included. So I am sharing this thought
today to show you by being "Optimistic" where it will lead you
too also. First "listen to" or play the video called "Optimistic"
by Sounds of Blackness. Focus on their words. I play it on my
ipod while walking on the treadmill and now the "lesson" for
today. When I first started walking on the treadmill after my
Stroke I could not do a lot. Maybe "1" minute at 0.5 miles

per hour. That is pedestrian for many but a chore for me. Yet this is where I started from. You see...they told my Wife and friends I would not walk again without "assistance". So I am truly blessed for sure. But God wants our best all the time too. We gotta do our part in the partnership. So I do the best I can. And now I can walk at "4 miles per hour" with an incline between 3-10. But this is not about the stats. It is about me staying..."Optimistic" and reminding myself how far I have come in this "new experience" called having a Stroke. We can move on in life yet we should never forget...either. So I went back to my "start point today" and for 10 minutes as a cool down I reminded myself. Because in this life it takes 3 things to keep "Optimistic". First...being willing to not give up on life. It does not mean you will not have bad days for sure. Second...remind ourselves what we have come through to reach this point in life. Third...you will always have struggles and be challenged in life. But by being "OPTIMISTIC" you are giving yourself a chance. It could be for any reason and you will decide that. I just wanted to share my story to help you see...its all good. It will be okay. But we have to do our part too. And that is to start somewhere. Decide and just go for it. But you gotta start...

BEEN THIRSTY FOR GOD

Have you ever been dying of thirst. I was thinking about it this morning while walking on the treadmill. Yes I was drinking a lot of water while exercising. My desire to drink water is real. That cool and refreshing - h2o. So after quenching my thirst I got back to taking those steps. Those steps turn into a Mile. Which turn into 2 or 3 Miles. But it starts with taking the first step to start. When I think about God it comes to me in all ways...not in bible form at all during my day. So today the message is on... Being Thirsty for God. All the time now. You see I have come a long way. He has been waiting for me for a while. He waited...and waited...and waited. And in the end he got me. Whether good and bad...it was always my choice. Sometimes good decisions are made. Other times bad decisions are. I have no one else to blame but tried too when it was a bad choice. When I was right it was all me even if I had help. Now do not think "trials and tribulations" disappear. They are still around every day. But with him by our side we get through them all. Sometimes with the scars to prove it. But having him "quench my thirst daily" is awesome. You too can get your thirst quench. It is a process for sure. And it never ends...so just take that "first step".

DISABILITIES TURN AROUND

> Some men came carrying a paralyzed man on a sleeping mat. They tried to take him inside to Jesus, Jesus answered them, "Healthy people don't need a doctor—sick people do. I have come to call not those who think they are righteous, but those who know they are sinners and need to repent."
>
> —Luke 5:18, 31-32 NLT

dis·a·bil·i·ty noun
- a physical or mental condition that limits a person's movements, senses, or activities. We are all sick in some way... I am not talking about the obvious which is present in people. Mentally and physical disability starts in "our minds". I know firsthand what it feels like to be mentally challenged. Pre-stroke and now because of this Stroke. Yet my mental capabilities now are what they are and I embraced them. But prior to the Stroke...I was in a "mental prison" also. My mind was not "focus on God" the way it is now. It was "focus on me" and my worldview - perfection...

ego...
material wealth...   .
self pride...
control...
spiritual forgetfulness...
sex...
fame...
jealousy...
and acceptance.

It happens to all of us. But now I see that these emotions and feelings were leading my life. Now I just "believe". God does not want me to "perform" or "do" anything in my life. He just wants me to believe - in him. And not depend on "my own understanding and knowledge of things"...but to just "lean on him". We can be cured by walking with God and seeking his help on a daily basis. So that you have a chance to embrace you "dis·a·bil·i·ty" too starting...today.

MERCY

> "God blesses those who are merciful, for they will be shown mercy."
>
> —Matthew 5:7 NLT

In reading this morning this verse stood out in my mind. Because everyone seeks mercy in some way or form everyday. When we make an error. When we answer wrong. When we are trying to address things we know nothing about but want to be relevant in the conversation. We all seek mercy then. But giving mercy is a bit of a struggle sometimes. Why...because "we can" receive it but not "give it". Why is that...for me its because "I had" put myself first. And you came second. When it should be the other way around. Because when I show people "his mercy"...I will get it automatically from God.

When I show this it is being humble. And with that "mercy follows" for both of us. It is really simple..."To receive mercy we have to show it first". Otherwise we are playing with fire. And when I play with fire...I get burned. Who wants that in their lives. Not me...

EVERY ONE PROBLEMS ARE DIFFERENT

This to us as "Stroke Survivors" it is time to give thanks again... to thank him for being "alive". Everybody is going through something these days...that is for sure. But when I consider my situation "I" have only 2 choices to make for the same question. What my FOCUS TODAY...on "me" or trying to help others help themselves. You see...we all have "our problems" which will not "magically disappear". That would be awesome...a "trick and treat" for sure. Whether great or small...when its "your problem" it takes on a whole new meaning. And hard for both parties...the ones trying to "help" and those in the "midst of struggling". While I cannot solve your problem I can share the burden...by listening first and trying to help you come up with "your own solutions". Because I know what it is like to lose everything too. So keeping your "HOPE"... which turns into a "BELIEF"...and then you have "FAITH" in something higher than yourself. I understand where you are because "I" used to think it was all "me" too.

A SIMPLE YET TRUE MESSAGE

> "Search for the Lord and for his strength; continually seek him."
> —1 Chronicles 16:11 NLT

I will listen and learn for sure. You see I do have a vision on things now. But before my Stroke I would "perform". Doing what "I" thought was right. And whether "right" or "wrong" was never enough. For me nor for you. But now by really trusting God...I can "be". You see we are all his "Masterpieces". Not sometimes but all the time in his view on life. So knowing this now the best thing I can do...is to "stay steadfast" in my focus. By concentrating on him and what he puts on my mind to do. To let him "show me" these days versus me telling him. Taking the pressure of "not doing it right" off myself. Following one simple rule..."be available to him". While a simple rule is to follow it is not easy to put in to practice at times. Because he knows better than each one of us what he wants done. So try to "be" ready. Because like me... you will never know when he will call on you. To "be" there for someone else...as their "next man up".

WE KNOW BOTH OF THESE

"Are any of you suffering hardships? You should pray. Are any of you happy? You should sing praises."
—James 5:13 NLT

There is a lot of suffering going on..."today". There are some with joy and peace..."today". Someone dealing with a problem..."today". With both of these emotions are on opposite ends of our spectrum...they "require the same solution". We "run and hide" or "think it us". You see if we are struggling or fearful..."HE" can handle it. When I think about all the joy..."HE" can do that too. "HE" handles it all for us. When we are "down and out" we tend to go into "a cave to be alone". When we are happy we think at times..."I did that by "myself". So the next time you are experiencing either one of these...the "HE" is God. Let him help because "HE" can handle it all... all the time. We just got to ask for his help whether "praying or rejoicing". And if you are like me..."I pray to rejoice". You see I have "LIFE" today...and you do too.

MY CHALLENGES REVISITED

When you have challenges in life you must make a decision of how to handle it. For me it was always "head on". It has been a while since my Stroke occured. But I am reminded of it all the time. Even today. My memory is bad. I cannot do anything with my cognitive skills. They come and go daily. My focus wanes. I can sit alone in my own little world...until disturb by others. My ability with counting numbers is getting better but at 50 I get confused and start over...again. All mental challenges are there but do you see them. I am sharing because I go through assessments all the time to "mentally to determine" when I am. I do my best always but my best sometimes is not good enough for them. But "their assessment" of me is what I deal with daily. Yet I look forward to it every day. You know why God woke up out of that coma. Because he was not done with me yet...and said so "in showing you" what his purpose is for me is now. The struggles associated with this Stroke can make life a living hell at times. If you take "that side on this stick". But for me I ask God for help each day. I asked him for his "mercy and grace". It is difficult for Lisa and others too. This Stroke is not easy for them as my Caregivers. We both are struggling "mentally" especially when physically things look fine. We are visual as people. We look at things from our own perspective because it is easier to do. It is safer too. Yet we all have mental things going on...in life. I just shared mine upfront. In doing so I am just saying to you..."It's Okay". We have challenges that people cannot see. I do and will for the rest of this life. So I accept these challenges and with God on my side..."I cannot lose". Remember this always "EMBRACE...WORK...DO YOUR BEST and PRAY". God is there and we just ask him for his help. I do it every day and he responds.

ADVERSITY INTRODUCES A MAN TO HIMSELF

ALBERT EINSTEIN

ADVERSITY

Adversity can be traumatic especially as a child. We have all been there. It was painful at times. It was hurtful too. But as we have to decided to take the next step. If we let it shape who we are now...that is on us. For me I take all my adversity in stride. All this adversity in my life makes me the man that I have become...today. You see now I can set my course on "new horizons" or just the same things as before. It's all up to me...and no one else. You have your own problems to deal with. They say "misery loves company". Well in this instance if we all are honest with ourselves there is something always that lurks in all our pasts. But how I deal with that adversity now shapes...but does not define me. Some of it I will deal with all my life. But the mindset is key. It allows you to deal with it or not. I am not attempting to take you and me through a psychological thing trust me. What I am saying is our mindset is a reflection to those around us. So I need Gods help every day because..."he knows it all". Yet he still loves us. He changes all those experiences into something that helps us now. You have just got to ask him for his help. It is so simple to keep the traumatic things in our lives today...but there is help too. I am siding with "Grace...Mercy and Faith". Sure its a big step for sure. Yet we can set new course with a "new horizons" and start next chapter in our "Journey".

CRUTCHES...WALKERS...CANES

> When Jesus heard this, he told them, "Healthy people don't need a doctor—sick people do. I have come to call not those who think they are righteous, but those who know they are sinners."
>
> —Mark 2:17 NLT

"Crutches...Walkers...Canes" support us while we get better. That is what they are for as we seek to be healthy again. But whether ever you are in that "Process"...know that it is a process for sure. So while we need them for the moment we strive to get off them too. And that is an individual process for sure too. It is so easy to say..."we need them" and some will agree. You see...our dependency on others is good when we need it but it is still up to "you". We have to "focus and concentrate" on raising that arm or leg a little higher. To speak and learn what words mean...again. While our families care...they do not truly know because "we" had the experience happen to us. But caring for us takes patience which can be tough at times...on them. Just remember that also. So let me help you both to understand this situation. We have to take a team approach to this uncertain time. Playing our part as we help each other to recover. Together we can take this on. Whether we "think" we are the "victim or a survivor" to "him" it is all the same. Because he and we know that "our crutches in life" are...both mentally and physically.

CHAPTER 2

"REBOOT YOUR MIND WITH NEW SOFTWARE" —A GAME PLAYED USING 6 WORDS

Strokes Explained "By The Numbers"

Why: *Many people think a Stroke happens in the heart, but it actually happens in the brain.*

6 WORDS TO SHARE

Just witness something interesting. Its using "6 words" to tell how you are feeling these days. What would yours be. No matter how dumb you think this is...its tell "your story" how you feel. And thats important. So go on and share them. I thought about using these...

"Crap deal wrapped in pretty paper".

"Experiences trump our knowledge every time".

"An emperor looking for a kingdom".

But when I really focus and concentrate on the task at hand I chose..."Today Living Best Life I Can".

AN IMPORTANT QUESTION

What can we learn from these challenging times in life these day during this pandemic. Do you "know"...Take a "guess". It is not about our cash...color...culture...community or circumstances. This pandemic only wants a relationship..."with us". That is all. It does not discriminate and takes on everyone. It does not care about "where you are in the walk" with the God of your choice. So like this moment in our lifetime..."he" only wants this one thing too. For us to "walk along with him" in our hearts and not our religious beliefs. Because those are only "walls" like this "virus" right now. Yet he seeks only one thing..."us living life through ACTION not WORDS".

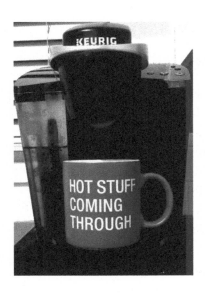

MORNING COFFEE

Woke Lisa up today with her morning coffee and a smile. We talk like we normally do for 30 minutes...my maximum. We always joke that between us we have a "single brain". Seriously though we talked about my bible study yesterday and what I learned from it. Truly to "Loving All". You see for me in those times where I am to "love a perceived or real enemy"...I have to lean in and trust God. He gives me a strength to listen to their story and not to interrupt them. You see in that moment of clarity God shows me..."myself". Because we all "only know what we know" in this life. So I stand up today as a REMINDER to say in my lifetime...I can "see you" in "me". It reminds me that I am not perfect and I show them off each day. My "imperfections" on full display like the Emperor did in the fable. But unlike the Emperor it's OKAY to show them to others. Read Hebrews 12:1-2 as I did to our group of "Imperfect Men" because it is a REMINDER..."TO RUN THE BEST RACE POSSIBLE BUT ONLY FOR...

TODAY". While we cannot solve anything without help. We can listen "without speaking" to each other so a story gets easier for them to tell. You see that "inconvenience" we are experiencing is for a reason. So that God can show "us" to us in other people. "Pardon the noise and the construction going on" is what "he" is saying at times shouting it out...over the hamster wheel we get on mentally. You see he is "constantly building" in and through us. Building in our "hearts" while "rehabbing our minds". With the purpose of showing us that in that moment of "inconvenience" we are still under "long term construction". So be grateful. Then passing this "act of kindness" along to others whether "a friend and foe". Stay encouraged and as always...be blessed.

I NEEDED TO CHANGE

Covetousness is not something we really talk about these days... so let me define it. According to Merriam-Webster Dictionary it is..."A strong desire to obtain some supposed good." Yes I know this well. Its really simple to explain to myself. "My needs" or "Gods desire" for me. You see when its my needs..."I" want it right now. But it was never enough...like a stomach searching to "be full". Do I "snack alone" or have a meal with someone else is what I am saying. I am trying to get full of the "snack"...but "a meal" is what I truly seek and need. So in these instances we continue searching for the next "great thing" in life to happen. Yet when we can let it all go...and just "rest in contentment" then it becomes God to work for us. Supplying us yet at his pace. You see his "desires" for us both to be "full". As a result of that I am not "dining alone" which allows me to FOCUS on changing my "I" to... "We".

"JESUS LOVES ME"

I was watching an episode of a show where the victim was wearing a t-shirt with a saying on it. Its made me think about something I would like to share with you. The person died. Any death is terrible. But as the detective said..."Whoever committed the crime did not love her that is for sure." Yet there are people ALIVE that do not think Jesus loves them. And due to this fact...there is a "Joy and Peace" they are missing out on. But it is not over until "The Fat Lady Sings". For those who have never heard that expression it means you have time until you die. You see until you die you can receive God into your life. I would not suggest this as we really do not know when we are going to die. I used to think when I was in my teens I would live forever. I was not worried about dying. Yet when I reached my 50th birthday I began to think about my mortality. In a humble way and actually glad God let me reach that age. Then at 56 years old I had a Stroke. Not just any Stroke but the kind that you do rarely come back to life from. Yet I am "here". Transformed by God my mind is at peace now. So it is my turn to share with others and hear their stories. What I am learning is there are a lot of troubled souls out there. They want to be heard but no one is listening. In some instances people are trying to yell over each other because they think that is a way to be heard. It is not...they just become a clanging cymbal or a noisy gong just created more noise as a distraction. All because they do not know or understand that "Jesus Loves" them. I did not understand it for a very long time. So we just got to ask our questions and seek him. And with that the saying on her shirt will become real for us...all. "Hazel" and I went for our walk this morning. It was a late start for us...5am. But as we walked..."step by step" today something was different. It was the same circuit that Lisa and I agreed on. Yet today it was full of "traffic". Which usually is not around but we did get a late start. It tossed "a degree of uncertainty" onto the two of us. As we walk together...we "talk to each other" also. And today we said this..."it will be okay". To keep our "FOCUS". To "KEEP GOING". To "NEVER STOP". Because our goal was simple...to get back "home" safely. You see there is a simple analogy here. We all have "traffic" in our lives. It can be a distraction...if we allow it to be. But you stay "FOCUS" and just stay steady. Because driving in "heavy traffic" is a lot different than when you are the "only one" on the road. It requires even more "concentration" than ever before. Because you like us... just "want to get back home" safely.

20 AT TIME...

You see I was watching this TV show and had this premonition. How this herd was going to drink water..."20 at a time". It is a reflection of our times of uncertainty "these days". Where we are limited in the people we can see. But this "piece of mastery on film" was done in the 1960s. Before this "uncertain thing started" or even was thought about. So the key of the story is "God" for me. He is the only one I know that has seen this all before. When he walks this earth as a "Man". Remember that all some of our ancestors did not drink from "his well either". His "living water"...as a collective was of offer. Some did and others did not. But he gave them all "sound advice" which many did not want to consider...back then and "now". And so today...he still wants all of us "drink" from his well. It is there...free for the taking. But remember to drink "20 at a time". That episode reflects our current times and the fact that everyone can still drink from his "well".

BACK IN THE SADDLE

"Dear brothers and sisters, if another believer is overcome by some sin, you who are spritual should gently and humbly help that person back onto the right path. And be careful not to fall into the same temptation yourself."

—Galatians 6:1 NLT

There are many temptations in life. Way too many to be listed for sure. All tempting us in some way. They do not seem to go away when we face them alone. That is why we need friends to help us...here and in heaven. So that we can help each other through these times. Because we watch and see with our own eyes the pain it causes. Yet at times we need that pain...because the way to grow. You see...if you never experience it how can you deal with it. Yet we all have painful memories...that we wish would go away. So my prayer for you today is for those memories to be relieved by God. "He" is the only one that can help even when we cannot see it. I have been there before. So in the meantime I will do my part too. To humbly and gently help you get back on your horse. That horse that will take you to the "Promised Land". Because you would do it for me...

BATTLE-FIELD COMMISSION

"From now on, don't let anyone trouble me with these things. For I bear on my body the scars that show I belong to Jesus."

—Galatians 6:17 NLT

I do not know about you but when "I fall or trip" occasionally... it produces a scar. Guess what...the smallest scars produce the greatest pain for me. But no matter what size of the scar is there pain involved. For "all of us". We do not get a choice either when the fall will happen or what that pain level will be. We all have what I called..."Battle Scars". While they hurt in the beginning they too will heal. Sometimes it takes a little longer than we want. The process of "making a scar" can turn into something else. You see we can choose to "let heal" or we can choose to "pick at the scab". You see whether mental and physical this "scarring process" happens in life. They never disappear but they do "heal" with his help.

Its A Choice You Make

"But when you give to someone in need, don't let your left hand know what your right hand is doing."
—Matthew 6:3 NLT

I am immune compromised. It means my emotional support dog "Hazel" and I walked at 4am...so that I am not in your way during YOUR DAY. It means during MY DAY...I am calling others to chat and see how they are. To care...to share by communicating with each other. So I ask one simple thing... yet some people find it hard to do. It is this..."Wear a mask." I do understand firsthand all mixed messages we are receiving for others. We swim in this "sea of information"...it is tough to tell what it really TRUE. Yet we all can stand at a "distance" because I cannot be right next to you. We save each other by doing this one simple thing. Yet it seemed to be a struggle as a "society" to do. This simple act of kindness "shows it all". That you really do care for your neighbor. In the meantime I will continue to do my part to wear my mask and keep YOU as safe in this "partnership" too.

SPECIAL TEAM OF LIFE

Hey when you make a block of a field goal or punt everyone like you. But what about the other times you are out there with no results. You are trying your best then too. Yet it is where you are successful that people actually pay attention to you. It is not the fault of the fans. They only know what they know. The ones that have played football will tell you that Special Teams are a necessary evil. You need it in your playbook. Sometimes the best players are not on the field for the "kick or punt teams"...but they are the same as a "starter". This is a chance to play in the game. It is like us being used by GOD. We are all capable. We are all wanted. All we have to CHOOSE to be "Available" no matter what our circumstances are. You would be surprised at the people that do not think they are qualified. Yet I can tell you this...we all can MAKE AN IMPACT one life...one person. So get set to go into this game called "Life". You are READY. You are AVAILABLE.

WAITING NOT IN OUR DNA

You see we like to hear "YES"...a bit disappointed with "NO"... the one we really cannot understand but need to hear is "WAIT". That when he yelled at us to..."trust him". There is more to come so we just have to be still for a moment or two. But waiting is not in our "Society of I"...but "YES" and "NO" are. True "happiness" comes from only one place. It is unconditional GRACE AND MERCY "shown" to us all each day. From the one who knows how to answer our prayers..."God".

ENCOURAGED ALWAYS

It sounds easy to do. Yet it is so hard sometimes. Though we all seek it at some point in our lives. In reality it does not happen enough or not at all. You know IF we can put ourselves in the shoes of the person thats "p*##**g us off" as they do. Extending the same "grace and mercy" to them that God extends to us. The question becomes our answer. You ultimately can encourage them. This is my example for you to consider. On Saturday I was with 2 friends. We meet at Chipotle in Dublin. That should have heightened my awareness anyway. The staff have "so many seconds to complete yours and my order". Well I finally made it through the "gauntlet of servers" and was at the last one. He wanted to finish my order with whatever topping I needed. I was trying to get it out. But was not quick enough for him. To make matters worse...I put my arm over the glass that separates them for us. Immediately he snorted to me..."Do not do that." I replied..."Do what as I was confused". He proceeded to tell me that I had placed my arm on the glass partition. He was right. But by then I was mad. I was sharing with him that I had a Stroke and the pace at which they wanted things for me I was trying to do. But it was not quick enough for them as they were working. I had to regain "my composure" at that point. Yes after a coupled deep breathes I took. And I what I did next was "the key" to my lesson for me. I put myself in his shoes. How they are trained to react to us as "Customers" in seconds. Well I need minutes to place my order. In the meantime their "process of serving" had come to a grinding halt. So truly understood his dilemma. Its made sense to me. Did not make it right. But I took the time to "realize his reality". And he did not know my situation because my "appearance" to him was like everyone else. I do not think he was even aware. But I was. So it was on me...to help him. I told him what a great job he and they were doing. It was the truth. I would not lie to him. And lets be honestly outside giving our orders to them...do we really care how they are doing. Not really. Yet from me came these encouraging words. Because we all seek and need encouragement. We can really thrive from it. But to give it is another story. One where we want to "pick and choose" who get it. The reality is EVERYONE NEEDS IT. Even when they do not think so or cannot tell you why our role is to "be nice" when they "don't want to play" at all. Because in the end we all need it. So I challenge you to encourage somebody today and everyday after...because we all need it.

FORTRESSES

"If you cling to your life, you will lose it; but if you give up your life for me, you will find it."
—Matthew 10:39 NLT

Life as we know it is a lot of things. Awesome at times. Yet the other end of the spectrum reveals not so good times. Fears... doubts...worry and other things can come into our minds in those moments. And with those things present we can start building a fortress around them. Where we not only believe them...but hold on to those emotions and feelings long term. When we look at the definition of a "Fortress" it means - a secure and strong place which can be defended from an attack. Well when we embrace these thoughts to the point of no return it a wrap. In fact no one else has to do anything to us. Because we will do it to ourselves. That is what happens in life at times. So we need to change our mindset. We need to "displace and replace". We have to give up our "old life" to receive the "new one". At that point we will start to see the same things differently. That we can overcome anything with God helping us by guiding our steps. We can see a way out from all that worries us. We receive a "PEACE" that we have never seen or had before. We all tried things our way for a long time. Yet "he" waits for us. "He" knows our burdens. "He" knows every way we can turn also. But we can only decide to come to him...as "he" patiently waits for us. It takes our "Fortresses" in our minds to dissipate...first. For a General means defeat but when we can do it it means...Life. Then and only then can we lead the life that God has planned for us.

FAILURES ARE BEAUTIFUL THING

I tried something new this morning for a change. You see... yesterday my friend Ken Thein asked a question. He asked me to "stretch myself"...not in the way of bending over to touch my toes. He meant "mental gymnastics" of flexing my mind causing it to "tear". To the point that we will get "stronger"...bending and flexing or twisting it at times. But it takes "practicing" so that when it is time to "play" you and I are ready. Well today I "prepared"...ready as I can be. My "practice" yesterday was perfect. But today...I "failed". I tried but was not successful as I wanted to be. But this "failure was awesome" because first I learned about myself and the added bonus is..."I tried". Even when I did not have to. So today the "best mediocre me" is present and accounted for. Yet I am okay with this because these "experiences" being taught from this book about "Surviving" are needed. It means some days you are going to..."FAIL". So just "try anyway". It is all you can ask of yourself. And no one else can fault you. You see there is beauty in everything when we "Failure". But you had the choice what your mentality is "today". To be a "Victim" or a..."Thriver". We just have to grab the..."right end of this stick".

GOD WISDOM VERSUS OURS

I was thinking about this... so bear with me. Because I did have a Stroke. I did not plan on it. It just happened anyway. People need to know that we all can learn from others. Because we do not know everything. We have the opportunity to learn from each other. But also know..."let students learn the lesson". And in the meantime..."the teacher sits quietly in the corner during the test". It is up to us to share at times by "being quiet". That is necessary in learning from a test. Letting people know that it is OKAY to learn at their pace...not ours. Because we all have be "there". Using "God Wisdom" versus our own gives us the chance to pass on the "lesson" that we want them to learn. Whether they know "God or not" is not relevant because he knows them by the name. And that is all we need to know as we sit quietly in "our corner". You see they have a lot of questions too...to ask of him. And like me he will reply in his own time by "showing them" also.

WE ARE LIKE VINEGAR...

I got a short one for you today. We all are like vinegar... progressing with age. To see it takes a while to get "fine"... in color and in taste. When we are younger...we are "clear" in our presentation of both. But as we get older we get "bolder" in our...taste. Yet both have something to teach each other. So the next time you can learn from someone older or younger than you...do it.

DEEP WATER IS NOT SO DEEP

"When you go through deep waters, I will be with you. When you go through rivers of difficulty, you will not drown. When you walk through the fire of oppression, you will not be burned up; the flames will not consume you."
—Isaiah 43:2 NLT

Well when you are a Stroke Survivor...it does not get much "deeper" than that. The uncertainty abounds all around you it seems. You are a "child again" in a grown body. How can I be James Thornton when I have no emotional attachment... to who I was before. But "I Am"...so now like me you have a choice to make. Get back "all that you can" or you can "die a slow death". It is not easy for sure but "my money" is placed on..."You" to get back all you can. People will look at you differently "now"...but "inside your head" your listening for their tone of voice. Yeah its seems like "hell" at times but we have only to do one thing. "Trust him"...because "he" has seen and experienced it all. So when you get up today and it all seems lost just ask him for his help. To guide your steps... and give your the strength to survive today.

Helping You Help Yourself...

"You will open the eyes of the blind. You will free the captives from prison, releasing those who sit in dark dungeons."

—Isaiah 42:7 NLT

I have been all 3 of these things in my life. Lets get that out of the way first. Because like you I am "human"...not someone unapproachable. Not like some people we know. The experiences I share with you are my own...not someone elses for sure. That is why I write to "show you my faults". So in reading this verse here is the deal. I was truly "Blind". Not in sight but in fact that I thought everything was in my control in my life. I was "Imprisoned" because of my mindset. Locked up with the key thrown away. I took the attitude of entitlement sometimes...in life and sports. I just wanted it all. Thinking that I worked hard enough but did not receive "my just reward". That is not my priority now. And I have sat in some "very dark places" over the years in my "mind". Do not want to go there but if I don't share that...I would not be telling the truth. You know what changes for me. Not my circumstances. Not my feelings or emotions. Not the situations that occur daily in life. The shift is how I see myself now. This simple and plain truth is..."God loves me". Even when I did not deserve it...he still did. This "Journey" we are all on is composed of "Chapters of...Then and Now". But one chapter written cannot affect the next one unless we let it. And finally being "alone in life" while it may seem strange to do is what most of us gravitated towards in our "bad times" versus the good ones. So knowing all this now allows me to say "let us be friends". "Care and Share" together. We all need a friend at some point as we write in our..."Book of Life". Try it... what do you have to lose.

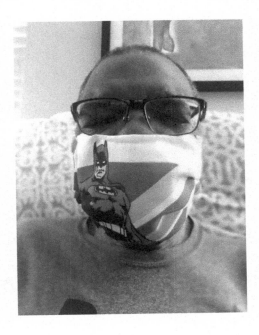

In Quarantine...Im Free

"I sit in silence" which is quite normal for me...yet I am not alone because of all the talking going on around me. So many voices all trying to be heard. Many have a lot to say...others offer only a single word. Yet all are looking for the same thing... to be heard with a shout or cry...but many cannot see of hear them. In my world of being "alone"...your identify for me comes from your image of what you see with your two eyes. Now I can speak once again...slow and steady...with a stutter or a slight pause. But you see "I AM thinking first"... because my ability to assume has disappeared with this Stroke. Now I reflected on my own life first...which is no joke. You see before ever saying a word...my goal is simple and plain... to offer you empathy for your circumstances...or situation because to examine my life first...to see we are both the same. But it is still "your story" to tell when you get ready too. But if I "think long enough" I can see myself in you.

CHAPTER 3
ITS YOUR CHOICE...NOT MINE

Strokes Explained "By the Numbers"

When: Every 40 seconds a Stroke occurs, killing a person every 4 minutes in the USA

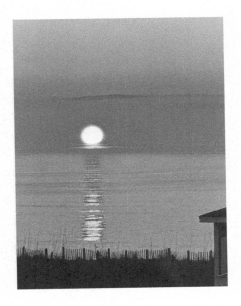

KEEP ON...KEEPING ON

"And since we are his children, we are his heirs. In fact, together with Christ we are heirs of God's glory. But if we are to share his glory, we must also share his suffering."
—Romans 8:17 NLT

I chose to dwell on what God promises during these uncertain times. I trust God to redeem all my pain to equip me to walk forward in faith and keep on fighting. Because I know what he has done for me when I did not deserve it. Yet he saved me from myself. Because all alone there was no one to lean on...so I did what I thought was necessary at that time. But now I can lean on him to get me things. Because he knows everything. Even though I cannot see or touch him...he is still there. And while I make errors in life he still loves me. And you too... "today". Because it is not how we start this race... but how we finish it.

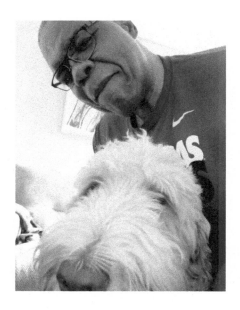

Its Crazy Out Here...

"Hazel" our puppy and I resumed our walks this morning. She is 1.5 years old...and well lets say "I am old enough to drive". As we got on our way I let "Hazel" lead. As she did... her focusing was on "losing her focus" then regaining it. The distraction of birds and other noises she heard...it is easy to do. A lot like you and me with other people. Those distractions we get every day in our lives. But I would get her to "sit" to get her back on her task. Taking care of me...as I take care of her. Because we walk together..."literally and physically" each time. And guess what she did not want to listen today. But that was okay...for I understood her dilemma. Because sometimes I want to do my own thing too. And God lets me. I am either "Walking the Walk" or "Talking to Talk" each morning with him. So by the time we returned home... we were in full agreement with each other. Because we were "walking together in stride" again. Like God does with us. He wants to "walk in stride with us" too. Yet sometimes we decide that we want something else. In those moments in our lives we think we do not need him. And he lets us think that way. Because he will wait "patiently for us"...unlike us with each other. Its so easy to get distracted or lose interest in someone else...especially in bad times. But when we focused on just "Listening" and keeping your "eyes on the prize" by not letting all the potential distractions "distract you today" you will "hear" the words being spoken to you.

LIFE

Romans 15:5 gives us the blueprint to living in this world but not being of it. We too can live in harmony with each other. It does not say our "race...culture...cash or religion" dictates where we stand. For "He" tells us to live a certain way. For me it is not playing God and being "judge... jury and executioner" in others lives. Hey I have problems running my own life. I am here to help people learn what they do not know. They are interested to learn more about themselves and in the process we both...help each other out. If they want to discuss God we can..."talking and sharing" what we know. But that is between God and them. And when it is time to make their choice about that...they will. I am only a part of the process to get them there. I just how them what is in my heart.

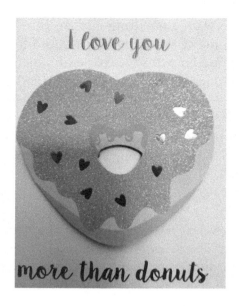

LOVE IN IT SIMPLEST FORM

"You are my LOVE!
You are my MAN!
You are my WORLD!
Only one man before you & that's GOD!"
—Lisa's inscription inside the card. Nothing else to say...

MY INVISIBLE BECAME VISIBLE

"In what way do you see invisible qualities"...statement not a question. For me it is through our dogs "Henry" and "Hazel". They love us both in a way that I can see how God wants me to "love". No matter what happens in our day they both love "unconditionally". So this morning as "Hazel" and I walked she jumped because something had frightened her...making her afraid. But in that instance of being afraid...I was there to comfort her. To let her know it would be "okay" and that we both are never alone as we are "out here" together. Whether

"Hazel and I" or "me and Him"..."his arms are constantly rocking away". At times..."slow and steady". Other times when we are in the midst of a storm. It does not matter because "he" is always "rocking us". So why "focus" on the circumstances of my Stroke. When God "uses me AND my circumstances" to help others. Yes these are uncertain times for us all. But its our choice to make about what to "focus" on. For me to see with my "own two eyes" the fact that he cares about me and you. But there was a time in my life that I would have "missed this moment". I was too busy with life...so I thought. So he "dimmed my use of my headlights" forcing me to "S-L-O-W D-O-W-N" and now "be a light" to others. Now I realize that "small things" in a career will lead to the "big picture" of life. I can see this now. It took me a while to learn this lesson. But "HE" will alway have time ⊘ to teach us as we learn the lessons in our own time.

MY BRAIN

We have two-sides to our Brain. One deals in our "Creative side". The other deals in "Logic". Like a symphony one is playing the "solo" while the other in the "background". And together in our beautiful mind the music of "thinking" is created. Each playing their part and nothing else. Well I walked through "a 3 month desert" after my Stroke because I could not FORGIVE and was RESENTFUL of you. But God spoke to my heart and changed me. Most of us are hesitant to resist change. But he always wins in the end. Because "he" showed me the way. The way forward. Because Gods love rained down on me when I could not love myself. Loving me so that I could love you. It's easy to love a friend. But how about someone you do not know...or an enemy. You see now I HAVE TO love that enemy as a friend too. Its not easy to do...yet it is. And while painful in the beginning...it will ease each time. Trust me I know both end of this stick. Because he allows me to remember back...sometimes way back. Do not ask me how or why...because I cannot remember. You see "I was that enemy" to someone before my Stroke. That is not a question...but a statement. And only you can decide to change your ways or stay the same. I write this with love and humility in my heart to address both sides of this coin. So you must decide too... when will you "remember".

MY SLIP SHOWING

> "And do not approach my altar by going up steps. If you do, someone might look up under your clothing and see your nakedness."
>
> —Exodus 20:26 NLT

When we idolize...we see "new and shining things" in our lives. Mine were "Work" and "Making money". With both there was never enough. And when I was satisfied the hunger came back...turning into more. But that is who we are. Its what we do. So God said he only wanted "his altars" made from earth. Not from "not from precious metals or any other man-made things" were to be used. Because they would only be significant for the person who built it...like myself. Like mine and your idol too. There will always be a new one. When we constructed them..."he" still will see truly how "naked we are". Yet in "our nakedness" he still loves us. But will we truly love him back. Because it's like I tell people all the time..."every once in a while my slip shows". Showing for all the world to see. And for me it is okay because I am "trying"...and he knows I am. But to "be naked"...well that is another story for another time.

NO NEED TO TALK

"My eyes will be open and my ears attentive to every prayer made in this place."
—2 Chronicles 7:15 NLT

God was having a conversation with Solomon...and said these words to him. No go-between or other person needed just the two of them together. As I read this verse today something struck me...like "lightning hitting the ground". What word "don't you see here". Its a big one yet "small in stature". Can you figure it out because it may take a while to see it "an action". Its the one thing we pride ourselves on at times. I can remember that I was a great talker back in the day...before my Stroke. But that has all changed now. I had no choice so I just listened. God was in a "teaching moment" even when I did not want it. But there "lies the secret" I want to share from my lesson learned you. See there is "POWER IN SILENCE". So that we all can "HEAR" each other. "SEEING" each other... through our own imperfection. "THINKING" before ever uttering a word...which is a good thing. It will lead us to "asking questions" versus "making statements". And with that...we can achieve what Solomon did. To work "together" to save...someone else from themselves.

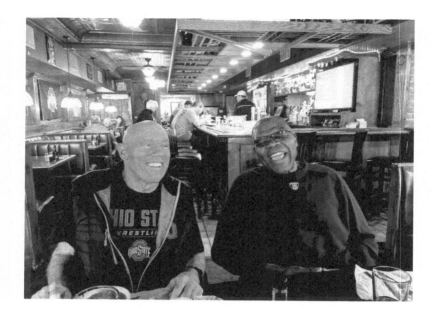

WALKING WITH A LIMP

"And I am convinced that nothing can ever separate us from God's love. Neither death nor life, neither angels nor demons, neither our fears for today nor our worries about tomorrow—not even the powers of hell can separate us from God's love."

—Romans 8:38 NLT

I actually slept last night for 2 hours. Then I woke up and started reading a book by a friend named Paul Nordman. The title..."Working In Us What Is Pleasing...To Him". It is a paperback and in short sections which make it easy to read. In Section 4 of this book there is an "Introduction of Jacob". I loved it because we all have been here..."the God of his father and ancestors but not HIS God". Man that struck me this morning like "lightning in a bottle". Because God gave me a "limp" too...to bring me home. With Drew all his life he thought he was not doing enough at times and his "performing" did not please God. But he would be given a "limp" also with "pain of war" as he served in the military. He saw many things from wars and like a "damn good soldier" he fought for us and our freedoms. Yet his "own freedom" he searched for after getting PTSD. But like me and you...God finally set him free. And all the rights of this world do not compare to his reward now. Because he is now in heaven helping serve people every day. So I write this morning because you have a "Limp" too and like us embrace it and be proud of it.

ONE WORD...ONE HECK OF A PROBLEM

"And whatever you do, whether in word or deed, do it all in the name of the Lord Jesus, giving thanks to God the Father through him."

—Colossians 3:17 NIV

Words...they have strong meanings. The same word can mean different things at times. And by a change of single letter in the sentence form...changes the whole meaning too. I know first hand the power of a word. I struggle daily with this fact of life. You do too. More than we both realize. Because words and how we use them can take something of joy and turn it into a painful situation for someone else. To others who are on the receiving end of it. We do not mean to...yet it happens. Sometimes we know exactly what we are doing...and it does not matter what the other person thinks. Because "we do not care". Because we are only concerned about "our feelings" not theirs. But really we do care. You see if we THINK before sending it in writing or saying a word the "sting" can turn in to a "prayer"...for them that hurt us and for ourselves. Because words are our "greatest weapon" that we are armed with. So treat them with care.

On My "Birth-day"

> "Is anyone thirsty? Come and drink— even if you have no money! Come, take your choice of wine or milk— it's all free! Why spend your money on food that does not give you strength? Why pay for food that does you no good? Listen to me, and you will eat what is good. You will enjoy the finest food."
>
> —Isaiah 55:1-2 NLT

I used to be..."thirsty and hungry". To find out about who God really "is". Because all I saw with my own "two eyes" is a world full of emotions and fears. Yet I knew there was beauty in the world too. But I could not see it. I was experiencing difficult times. I do not see the "brighter side of life". God why are you not taking care of things for me. Well I had the wrong end of the stick. I could not see all of the beautiful things because "my mind" did not allow it. To change my view and focus on such things..."then". But now I see and understand the beauty of every circumstance. "We" have to seek. "We"...have to believe in something. "We"...must put our trust in something bigger than us. I still have questions and seeks answers but with a different mindset "now".

Our Love For Each Other

> "If I could speak all the languages of earth and of angels, but didn't love others, I would only be a noisy gong or a clanging cymbal."
>
> —1 Corinthians 13:1 NLT

Lisa and I have a RESPECT for each is one of our cornerstone principles. It is paramount whether living alone or together with someone. We all want it. But do we give it freely away. You see we all live on this earth together. We have a daily choice to make from our hearts. We can have our differences for sure.

We do. Yet we all want to be heard but sometimes listening and hearing is tough. Yet is what we expect for others. To... LISTEN. Now people tell me I am different from before my Stroke. That I am truly HEARING them. That I am NOT INTERRUPTING them as they speak. God took me through "3 months" of silence. All I could do was...LISTEN and was amazed by the stories I heard. They knew their "secrets were safe" with me. Not being able to respond or answer them...I heard it all. So I just took it in stride and it why I respect you today. It is due to the fact that I truly care about what you say..."today". As a "mute" I was shown things about our lives. Everybody has "someone or something on their chest" to talk about. Then I could not reply. Now I chose not to reply as we talk. So I extend a challenge to you today...RESPECT someone not in your circle of friends. Start there...you may be surprised what they tell you too.

REJOICE ON A RAINY DAY

> "Sing praises to the Lord who reigns in Jerusalem. Tell the world about his unforgettable deeds."
>
> —Psalms 9:11 NLT

Today my sidekick "Hazel" and I walked and it started to rain. I decided to press on walking of course and it was great. And while a little wet there was only one thing I could focus on..."Why could I do this...today". It is because I am here... Alive. Thankful because of "his" grace and mercy on my life. "I can"...speak with a voice again. "I can"...count up to 30. "I can"...write again. There are more "I can" in my life... more than ever before. While they may seem small in size some would say...they are "great in stature" for me. Because now my "small words and ways" are impactful to others. But it all started with "him" saving "me" by waking me up from my coma. He wanted you to see for yourself one of his

"unforgettable deeds". You see we all have a "story" to tell...
its may seem small. But great things come in small packages.
So be willing to share it...and watch what happens.

"ROOM" FOR YOU TOO

> "My Father's house has many rooms; if that were not so,
> would I have told you that I am going there to prepare a
> place for you?"
>
> —John 14:2 NIV

I recently wrote on being "Patient" and how it is a choice
that we have to make daily. "To be...or not to be" is truly the
question we face each day. Some days are better than others in
practicing this. But as he said..."there are more rooms than we
can ever go into" in his house. It is all because "HE LOVES
US ALL". Before my Stroke at times I would "sit still and
wait" but not very often. I was on the go all the time. Asking
you a question but then..."answering it for you" too. Then
I suffered this Stroke because while my body was in shape...
my "brain was not". That experience has taught me that we
all have a voice. It is our choice whether we listen and hear
each other or not. You see I still have "1" talent to use now
a special gift called the..."Gift of Encouragement". Which
means I listened first all the time now. So when you think
about this verse today...know that God has made room for
you too in his house.

TAKE THE TEST

> "Blessed is the one who perseveres under trial because, having stood the test, that person will receive the crown of life that the Lord has promised to those who love him."
> —James 1:12 NIV

Day 2 of the..."new normal". While I cannot tell you what that is. I can definitely tell you that is happening. For everyone on this earth...at the same time. While what we are experiencing may not look the same... It is all the same worldwide. "Uncertainty" and "unsure" about what happens next are the 2 things dominating conversations being held around this world. And rightfully so. These are uncertain times. They make us feel unsure about what we are seeing. Whether about life...school... what to eat because store shelves are empty or something else happening in your life...it is a really scary situation. Real life. The real deal. But know what...we are all standing up and taking this test and will receive our reward at the end. But not any reward for sure but the one God promises us. You and I. Because while we cannot answer all the questions we have right now - he can. And while it may take days or months or years to see the answer to these questions...we only have "today". Actually..."this moment". So do not worry about tomorrow. It has its own problems for us. We are not promised to see it either. But "today" we woke up and that is a blessing. If you are concerned about things...you should be. But take comfort. We just have to keep our eyes on the "real reward".

WALKING A TIGHTROPE

> "I could ask the darkness to hide me and the light around me to become night— but even in darkness I cannot hide from you. To you the night shines as bright as day. Darkness and light are the same to you."
>
> —Psalms 139:11-12 NLT

I "walked a tightrope" at times. Walking in both darkness and light. My darkness represented all things..."I" wanted. While the light represents...what I do for others. Yet in my darkest moments I did not think God heard me. Crying and pleading because I thought I was "alone". But he heard me. He had not gone anywhere. But I did at times...to be in control of everything. Yet while I was crying out...he already had answered me. But the things he was telling me to do...was not to "my liking". So I continued to do things my own way. But now I realize that in the darkest moments...I must change my ways. And still see that I have a choice to make...today. I just got tired of "walking around in the dark"...thinking I was alone. We choose to go it "alone" or have a "partner". But for my "walking my tightrope"...get tiring.

A "REALITY CHECK"

> "God blesses those who are poor and realize their need for him, for the Kingdom of Heaven is theirs."
>
> —Matthew 5:3 NLT

We know that people are..."Poor". There are "poor circumstances" which we have gone through. There are "poor choices" we all have made in life. But think about this...to see we are all "poor" in the same way. While I thought you were "poor"...I am too. Not in things of this world because they will always "come and go". But "pride" and "money" were two of my favorites rides on "the playground". But then God slowed me down to where I could notice him. He gave me an insight.

Which is..."I am poor now" in every way. It is a reality that I did not count on getting...but so glad I did. You see on this "playground" every day is like riding the "see-saw". "Up" one a day and "Down" the next. It is the world we live in now. But if we change our mindset and give up control whether "up" or "down" that day...know that "he" will get us through it. Not because of who we are in life. "He" stands for showing us "his" love" through grace and mercy to meet our needs.

EMPATHY IN AN IMPATIENT WORLD

We are impatient. We want it now. We want it all..right now. But what we need to do is...slow down. Slow to the point of listening. You see if our mouths are open and we are talking too fast. So fast that our mind is not engaged before we finish our sentence. And that is not what is needed. We need to share our mercy and grace with each other. You see..."I Am You". And..."You Are Me". Empathy is what we all need the most. Because we all are on the same "Lake"...just in different "Boats". In the same "Storm"...make no mistake about this fact. And with that "empathy" we have a chance to listen and learn...about something other than our needs.

COMPLAINING

Today Lisa and I attended a great worship service then decided to go to brunch at our favorite place. As we sat chatting about the sermon she threw me for a loop. She said this, "We all complain about something in life." I asked her to repeat that statement to be certain I had it right. She did and I did. I thought about it long and hard. She could tell that something was going on "inside of my head". I stated then I was going to write at some point. I had to "think about it" first. You see I used to be one to complain a lot back in the day. Now it is just one..."We do not have enough LOVE in this world." I was told in my teen years years if I was going to complain I had to come up with solutions also. So in keeping with that premise is what I have come to learn now...

- "I LOVE MYSELF because GOD LOVES ME".

- "I LOVE PEOPLE even when they cannot or will not LOVE THEMSELVES".

- "I LOVE MY NEIGHBOR as I do myself."

Yes we all can complain. It is our nature and what we do. But when you find a solution to put into practice...you resolve the complaint. I resolve my complaint with 3 simple words..."I LOVE YOU". So when you complain today...think about how much we have in life to be thankful for first.

ACTING ON... "THE WORD"

"Then Jesus said to his critics, "I have a question for you. Does the law permit good deeds on the Sabbath, or is it a day for doing evil? Is this a day to save life or to destroy it?"
—Luke 6:9 NLT

Many people see Saturday and Sundays as the time to attend a church service. And they are correct if you "believe"...in something bigger than yourself. But just because we go to church and read "The Book"...thats only half battle won. You its easy for us "to preach" to others. But it so much better to "show them"...our love. Because "they" need that more than anything else. As we do. You see while "Reading is fundamentally". Our actions toward them is all they need to see. We too have a chance...save a life or destroy it. Because walls or a building does not make who we are..."now". It because of "who" lives inside of us. Therefore we are the "church".

CHAPTER 4
NOT THE END...JUST BEGINNING

Strokes explained "By the Numbers"

Where: It can occur at any time. The warning signs are called F.A.S.T.E.R. Go to an Emergency Room within the first three hours.

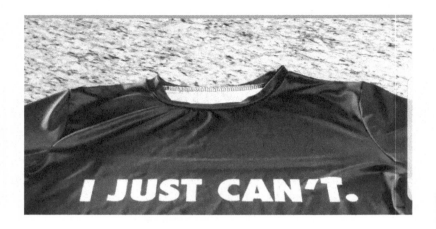

CAN'T ISN'T A WORD

> "What do you mean, 'If I can'?" Jesus asked. "Anything is possible if a person believes."

> —Mark 9:23 NLT

This one is short and sweet. But how sweet it is. As a Christian I had a duty. Not to brow beat you or make you feel like you need Christ in your life. My duty is simple. Let you "SEE" how God works in my life. Let you "SEE" I have my issues too. Let you "SEE" how God works on my behalf because what I came up with is not the answer. Not part of the time but all times. And share my story with you. Then it is "SHUT UP" and "LISTEN" to "YOU". Listen to your success. Listen to your failures. Listen to your questions about life - career, personal and spiritual things. "YOU" decided on what to tell me. "YOU" choose the order. "YOU" choose when to tell me. You see only then are we starting building a "RELATIONSHIP" with each other. This all occurs because we only know what we know in this life. Sometimes we think we are good. Sometimes we are searching. But wherever you land on this chart we can always learn more. So we will do more..."TOGETHER".

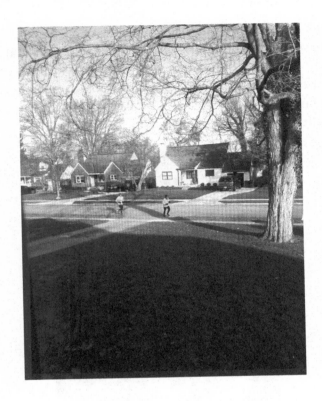

1 FOOT OR 100MILES STILL IS THE SAME

I took this picture and wanted to share with you. It our son Pierce and Albert a cousin of ours. They are running for a Cause today called..."CancerFREE Kids". But what is different is there is no cheering right now. I am certain it will come later on. So I went outside as they rested for the 10 minutes they get each hours to tell them how proud I am of them. When people are not around and tough times are upon us..."that is when it counts most for no other reason than you try your best". It is in those moments when there is no one there to cheer us on...that when "our determination" has to drive us. All of us have these opportunities to try. For me it is trying to doing 1.5 mile loop walking. For so many it is raising an arm or a leg higher than yesterday...which seems like "running" because of the effort it takes. So today like Pierce and Albert did run your best race knowing it was a "100 mile marathon and not a sprint". Slow and steady wins this race today. Did I mention that we talk that day at 4am and then they went on to finish by running the best race possible. Like we do in rehabilitation.

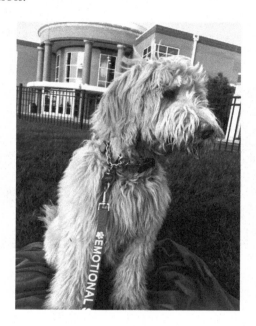

TWO DOGS LEARNING THE SAME TRICK...

"Focus...Focus...FOCUS" I have to do this every day. I have no choice...its not an option. I have a story to share. Our dog "Hazel" walks me around on a "set course". She is a Labradoodle puppy about 1.5 years old. I am a 58 years old man. So getting in our walk first thing in the morning is key for our health and the pursuit of happiness. During our walk though the neighborhood...we concentrate on one thing. To "focus" on each other and no one else. And guess what happens at times to us both...we lose our "focus". Not at the same time...which is the blessing. She gets distracted by the lone squirrel going between trees or by bird chirping and even an occasional fire hydrant. But I just tell her to "re-focus" and she immediately snaps back. And me...I lose my focus too. The problems of the world are mine too. That is the reality of life. We can "color it" anyway we want but if not careful...you will lose "your focus" too. It can happen at "drop of hat". So getting back "re-focus" is our key. As "Hazel and I" do each time we walk together. After we are done I always tell her..."You did well. You are getting better each time. Keep it up." And guess what...God saying those exact words to me and you too.

BITTERNESS IS DEADLY

> "You gave me life and showed me your unfailing love. My life was preserved by your care."

> —Job 10:12 NLT

I had a setback. Not another Stroke. Just a setback... And while I sat last night and thought about it. I forget the one thing which means more than any setback. I am here because of one thing..."God". Like Job from the bible my disappointment consumed "my fire" also. So I can be mad and bitter. But bitterness is deadly. Because it gets us down and we can wallow in our mud...to a fault. Its my choice to make every day. My choice that day was to celebrate this life that God gave me back. You see we all will have setbacks in life. It is how we choose to respond that really matters. And no matter what the setback is...I move on. Singing and dancing as I celebrate the one and only thing that matter...my life. Because God loves a "Winner"...and we have all "Won" in his eyes. Like Job we too will receive our reward in the end...if we choose to hang in there also.

> **Focus impacts perspective. If you want to see from Jesus' perspective, then you need to stay focused on Jesus. Today, let's learn how to do that.**

REPAIRING MY ROOF

Today they are still working on replacing our roof. I struggle with "noise in general" because of my Stroke. I am at home every day due to my Guillain Barre Syndrome. So "People 👥 and Things⛏" are always making sounds because they all want "to be heard" in my world. But I figured if God sent his "Son to walk this earth as a Man" performing "miracles after miracles" yet it was not enough for us. So he made the ultimate sacrifice of letting his Son die on the cross...for us. Throwing all of our sins into the "Sea of Forgetfulness". Which means if he "struggled" then and I can now. With "Hazel" lying at my feet and with God helping both of us with all the sounds around us it inspired me to share with you this writing. You see...there was a time that I did not "listen completely" but "he" still loved me. I had "no choice" in the matter. But now although I can see the "errors in my ways then"...I still can help others now. It is like we say..."Only God can save. We just want to be a part of that process". And like our roof this week...I needed to be "repaired too".

OUR HEALTH...TODAY

Health problems...hopefully you do not have any. And if you do my hope is that you make the best recovery possible. But the true "crisis" right now for all is our...."Mental Health". Its taking hits like never seen. Because no one could or did... predicted this "global pandemic". All of us...no matter what we do are experiencing something. Mine is hoping people know "that we all a truly are our brothers and sisters keepers". And they understand the life the saved is someone else...mine. We all had problems before this even started. But now a virus has been added to it "sprinkles" with our issues of relevant topics and "topped off" with a cherry. For what we have made ourselves quite a sundae. It is filled with anxieties and fears...one more powerful than the other at times. But like that Energizer Bunny we see on TV...we all have to get up and stay up. Not an easy thing or simple to do at times. You see I depend on a lot of people daily...to help me through this thing called life. So the lesson today is simply this. Let go of whatever dictates your life. Let this go and "get it off your back". Because our Mental Health is a key to walking out a good life...waking up and looking forward. Not feeling stressed nor lonely. These "pains" could be just starting or have been around for awhile. Feeling alone can make you think about all the "hits" you took today. Whether from our "psyche perspective" or physically...it will affect us both. So seek help...because that is a choice too. Put your best foot forward or suffer...it is totally up to you. But I suggest taking the first step to let go of our "pride and ego thing." Then you are truly making room to get the help deserved and needed. Finding answers for what is troubling you and getting the required counseling. If you choose to do nothing but work it out alone...will be in "self quarantine". And with that "isolation"...no one to help you deal in that outcome.

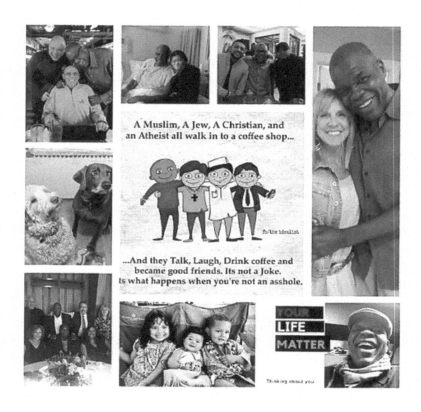

"OUR WORLD"...

We all share the same feelings and emotions in societies around the world. "We are...all the same in my world".

MY COMMAND VERSUS HIS

"This is my command—be strong and courageous! Do not be afraid or discouraged. For the Lord your God is with you wherever you go."

—Joshua 1:9 NLT

I used to be a "Commander"...back then. Being in charge. Taking control. Leading people. But these days what I realize is this Stroke happened to me and now I am "not in charge" of anything but my own life. I have "no control" over anything except me. And this last one is most important and key to me surrendering and being led now by something other than myself. You see I am the same man that I always was...but there is a difference now. I can see the "blind spot" of being stressed for so long in life. To realize these are stressful times for all of us. But God gives us HOPE in this verse because "he" cares. So receive this gift and then apply it today in your life. We already know what stress feels like. So you have nothing to lose in trying this new approach to being much happier.

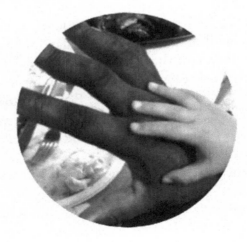

GRATITUDE FOR EVERYTHING

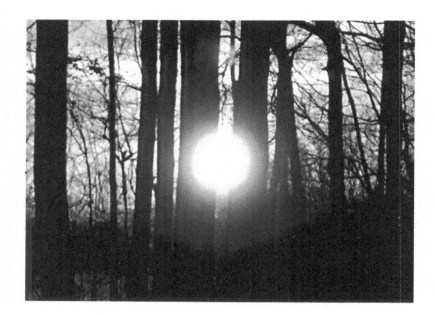

Sunshine For All

Yes its sunny outside and it makes staying inside our homes really hard. Easter and Passover are coming this weekend also. And to top it off you may be experiencing "cabin fever" at the moment. People picketed yesterday for the first time in a fashion that says they want "their rights" back. Back too a normal life that has been taken away for now. Yet it is a short-sighted view in my opinion. Because I too want my rights back...to do things outside of the house yet cannot. Being outside without fearing the unknown would be great. I could do the following activities...

To have the chance to meet up or fellowship with others again...

To go to get a haircut which I need without my fear...

To have a "beer and lunch" with friends or attend something outside of my home for a change. But I know why these things will not happen for me today. Because "I" replaced my thoughts and feelings with "You". I will not allow myself to think about me. While as tempting as it sounds for sure the temptation is not worth taking. I want to at least try and give it our best "shot"...pun intended. You see "this thing" we are all dealing with knows "no borders". Does not care about our nationality but we do. It does not discriminate. Yet it does kill. Best case is we get sick...and recover at some point. So while I understand the "cabin fever" you may be experiencing. I wanted to share this with you...the lives you are saving are yours and mine. That is definitely worth me giving up "my rights" for the time being. Because I LOVE you as I do myself. While it is biblical written...putting it into Action is the reality of our times. It does not matter whether we know each other or not. Because we are both the same in this instance. This reflects the ultimate Easter message that I can deliver to you personally...but at a safe distance.

THE TRUTH...HELPS NOT HURTS

"To do what is right and just is more acceptable to the Lord than sacrifice."
—Proverbs 21:3 NIV

In this storm called life...we all are doing the best we can. It may not seem this way to others sometimes. Because the problem is not "mine" but "yours". But I must think back... way back or to yesterday. Because that same problem I had then..."you" have today. And whether you are aware or not saying this truth helps us both. It is painful...to both sides. It hurts. Yet the disaster waiting to happen can be avoided or reduced. By saying nothing I am really saying..."I care about you not just now". Because I was taught by my Mom...and oh what a lesson learned about LOVE. It must show it to you... through ENCOURAGEMENT as by CHALLENGES YOUR THINkING and offer that EARNEST ADVICE which we all needed. All done in a loving and humble way. It is how we share this EARNEST ADVICE that counts most. It is not a command. There is no need to "preach". It just complicates and confuses things. I say this because it is true. I remember back...to when I did not want to hear this either. I have learned how to "show" the same things I receive in those moments. Using compassion as I listen to your story of "how and why". Speaking when it time too but as a "friend". A place of caring for them. And only then can I offer the advice...like I received when I did not understand. Helping me to save myself ... "from me". They say..."The truth hurts". It may or may not at that moment. Yet by sharing with each other we accomplish "2 things". First we are acknowledging that mistakes will be made in life. And then by sharing our stories you can decide what is best for you and your situation.

FOCUS, FOCUS, FOCUS

People who know me will tell you this... I have a "one-track mind" these day. I used it every day to its potential. Those around me can easily be distracted. For many reasons. With many things going on in our lives...its easy to lose concentration and your focus. When that happens we can get lost. Losing in our "good mind". Losing focus on "our goals". Yet God can and will anchor us...no matter what. When we are struggling and need a port to call our own he is there to anchor us as we ride out the storm. To get us to a place of calmness. So that we can face one or more storms on our horizon. I have had many storms in my life. Some I got to use God as my "anchor". Yet many times my boat was "tossed by the waves". You see my anchor back then was "me"...my pride or jealousy and anger. My "control of things" is used as "my weight of choice". But even then God helped me survive those storms also.. Because he could...he would. Even though I could not see him there. Yet he was as always there protecting me. To pick me up and dust me off telling me to get back into the game. So when your little voice inside your head says...why are you trying so hard. You can answer back with..."I have nothing to lose." Because this "game" called life waits for no one.

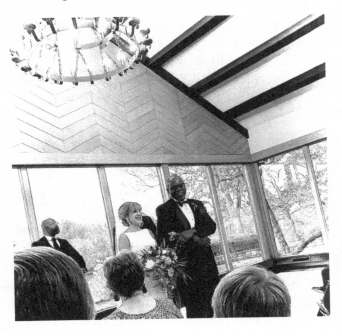

Our Marriage Yesterday

> Faith shows the reality of what we hope for; it is the evidence of things we cannot see.
>
> —Hebrews 11:1 NLT

We were married yesterday and it was definitely a joyous occasion for the both of us. Sharing it with people from far and wide was wonderful. They came from all part of the globe and religious backgrounds did not matter. For Lisa and I it was time to make a pact that is sealed in stone to each other. But sharing the day was most important for us. As my best man Mark Riley and I sat this morning recounting the day. From his standpoint from our vows to each other to meeting so many people last night he said it was "truly epic". I am going to go with his perspective on things. It does not matter whether you attended or could not make it..."we love you". All people make the world go round. All backgrounds. All races. All religions. Our faith is truly in what we cannot see... but believe in our hearts. Our faith leads us. It lets us believe in you. Even if you doubt yourself we still believe in you. Because we are blessed by people believing in us "from all over the world" this day.

HEAR THIS...

Hey this message...its needed. But as my Reverend says..."you may not want to hear it". It is this..."If we do not have a diverse view about things...we cannot display empathy to others". Which is the "Mercy and Grace" we receive daily. Aware of things from only our point of view and have no faith in "anyone but ourselves"...is probable and possible. It reflects what "you" believe in. But our world is a diverse fabric. It does matter your color and cash and religion in this instant. Because that diversity of thoughts makes us who we truly are..."messed up and in need of help". Just because we do not like to hear that about ourselves does not make it right. We must come alongside to share what makes each "one of us"...tick. To get to know a person so that we realize we have more in common than what seems to "separate us"...at this point. There is only one "judge" who can judge us all. But I find it interesting that we can judge each other in an instant... without reflecting on our "own life". It occurs because we choose too without conversing first.

HAZEL TAUGHT ME TODAY

"The seeds of good deeds become a tree of life; a wise person wins friends."
—Proverbs 11:30 NLT

I truly believed this verse...but was shown to me today. We walked our normal route this morning like we always do. But there was something different about today. You see...for the first time "Hazel" and I walked in step from the first to the last..."step-by -step". We normally talked to each other. Yet today...we both spoke in silence to each other. We enjoyed taking in all the wonderful things going on around us...squirrels jumping and rabbits hopping all around us. But we were enveloping in our silent walk...together. By our last step she had shown me that we are..."in this thing" for life. You see I never wanted a Stroke but had one. It is not like you wake up one day and decide your are going to have one. The days of uncertainty were real and true. Yet I had a choice to make from the first day. To "give up or fight like hell" to get back something...anything. It has taken a while but what I receive is "life"...is it glory. But took me getting out of my own way... to let him do his thing once more. Showing me "Grace and Mercy" of bringing me back physically and mentality. While awaken me spiritually this time showing me that "I am never alone". For God does not make mistakes...but we do. He has demonstrated a love that only "Hazel can duplicate". It is unconditionally with a little humor sprinkled in. You see...G-O-D spell backward its D-O-G.

MY NAME IS JAMES...

Today I read from the Book of James. Basically about faith and our works in life. I will focus on this though...his questions to us. For by him questioning himself he displayed his bravery. In the light of realizing his faults he wondered about things. Brave enough to ask us all questions related to... his faith. Because our faith has to be displayed for others to see. Because we forget that part sometimes. You know what I mean...the part about everyone seeing. The "Display" for all to see from the unsure through to a fellow Christian. Show all in a loving and humble way. A way that says I love you. Not sometimes but all the time. Not when we want to but always. Yet we have to seek and accepted this love first. Then we can focus on giving it away. Maybe you have bills you cannot pay. Workers you have to let go. Worries and fears about the future. Or just wanting to go outside without worry. There is a long "laundry list" of things for sure because everything is fair game for discussion. But it all boils down to one thing. A simple and true down question. Not in "man"...but a higher being. What you "believe in" I will accept. But I can "show you" my God...firsthand.

A "RIGHT" FOR ALL...

Written January 6ᵗʰ 2021 the day "our US Capital" was taken over.

> "But to all who believed him and accepted him, he gave the right to become children of God."
> —John 1:12 NLT

Our "CHURCH with its RITUALS" was violated today. All of us saw it with our "own eyes". You see we all want and seek "RIGHTS" in ways that offer us something better...we think. We see it as..."PRIVILEGE". Something "SPECIAL" that we need and want. A "RIGHT" to let us move like we want to in life. To seek what its "RIGHT-fully ours". So if this is really true why do we not accept the greatest "RIGHT" of all. The one that give us..."freedom". The one that "can save us" because we "canNOT" save yourself or anyone else. The one that offers us "strength" at our "weakness times" in our lives. It does not matter what you have. Cash is not needed. Culture does not matter. Religion does not matter. Circumstances need not to apply either. You see I used to "fight for RIGHTS" too...for myself and others. But now I have the "GREATEST RIGHT" of all. Being a child of "God". It came with a price that has been already paid. My story is for his use now. But it is still your choice to make also. Because he will pursue us by waiting patiently for us. Yet you and I have to want this "RIGHT" and all that comes with a price tag too.

PIGPEN BY A NOSE

"Publish his glorious deeds among the nations. Tell everyone about the amazing things he does."

—1 Chronicles 16:24 NLT

When I read this verse it makes me think about my own life. Its reminds me that HE knows all of my struggles. Before my Stroke...and after. HE knows all. My worries. My pride. My feelings that would always get in the way. Yet he still sought me out...ME. When faced with this decision he decided it was ME. When HE did not have too do a thing. I still would by struggling today. But I do not anymore. It is something that I did not want to recognize before my Stroke. Yet now I do. With the same PRIDE I had before but now it shows outward. So people can now SEE for themselves so "preach it" is not necessary. Because that was not the way to reach me either. But showing it now is a totally different story. You see...I am "Pigpen". You know from the cartoon character from "Charlie Brown" lore. You have the main character Charlie Brown. He his trusty friend named Linus. Lucy is his shrink. There are many characters including "Pigpen". I am this character because of all my sins and struggles. Whether good or bad all are now on full display. For you to see for yourself. God helps me with these every day...all day. My "dirt" can be seen by HIM and by you. Yet I still choose ME...as he knows all. So it's okay...it really is to show your true colors and feelings. Its okay to truly say you are tired or alone and want help. But it is not okay to "decide" that you can do it by yourself. You see..."we all have a pile of dirt to play in".

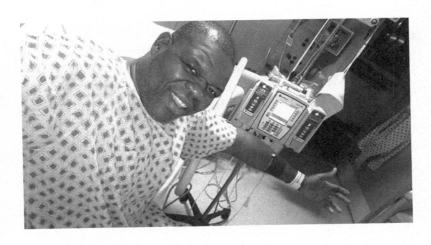

SURVIVING IS A CHOICE

"I don't know what your destiny will be, but one thing I know, the only ones among you who will be really happy are those who have sought and found how to serve."

—A. Schweitzer

I want "6 Words" to describe how you feel. The question is..."How does my Stroke help you in your life journey." It is not about me at all. Only YOU can tell me what is in your heart and in your mind. You see HE brought me back after lying on my bedroom floor for 20+hours. When found by friends I was transported to Riverside Hospital here in Columbus Ohio. While sleeping I went to a place unlike any other... to see "HIM". No "angels" or loud talking from him. But in a whispering voice he said..."You are going back because I am not finished with you". While I was in my nirvana back at the ranch it was not good news being shared. Doctors told Lisa and friends there was nothing they could do medically. You see I had past the timeframe to use TPA a drug used to help the brain heal. "IF" represented a BIG WORD at that moment in time. "If" I survived and woke up it would truly be a MIRACLE. "If" I regain consciousness at worst I would

71

be a "vegetable". Best case scenario I would be rolling around in a wheelchair or on a walker for life. So when I woke up that fateful day God had changed me. Not a physical change...but mentally. My "weaknesses now" would be on full display... every day. To show you "his strength" through the "mercy and grace" he gave to me. Walked "through in a desert" for the first 3 months by being "mute" and silent. I could hear you and others from Day 1 but could not answer back. So God was just fine tuning my ability to HEAR your voice. This gift of PEACE I cannot describe. But it took something tragic for this to occur. But we all are "Survivors" of something if we think about it. But I want you to "Thriver". That is my best wish for your family and caregivers... and YOU too.

A LAUGH TO SHARE

"For God, who said, "Let there be light in the darkness," has made this light shine in our hearts so we could know the glory of God that is seen in the face of Jesus Christ."
—2 Corinthians 4:6 NLT

I have been told that I have a great laugh. One that makes people smile...no matter how they are feeling. Its because its genuine and authentic. In laughing it must really be funny. Yet I can "see" something about "you" in myself. No closer...a little more...now stop. What you see in my JOY for life...now. And while I want to think before my Stroke I had joy...it's not like now. Does not compare because of the simple reason I could not find it everyday back then. God then took away something yet gave it back to me...LIFE. What a wonderful thing to receive back from him. So for right now I will be your "beacon on light". I can do this for you because it was done for me. And you just need it right now. A break from life in all its glory and challenges. To laugh and smile if only for a minute. But in that 60 seconds we can escape...together.

CHAPTER 5
USE UNTIL WE ARE TOGETHER...
AGAIN

"Dear children, let's not merely say that we love each other; let us show the truth by our actions."
—1 John 3:18 NLT

LIFE IN ALL IT GLORY

"This means that anyone who belongs to Christ has become
a new person. The old life is gone; a new life has begun!"
—2 Corinthians 5:17 NLT

I depend on everybody...each day. You...yes you. It is my new
normal and I love it. I know the good and bad situations you
see...because I also did these things to others in my life...not
intentionally. But you know what...God still loved me...even
when I could not love myself enough. So while the world
its in a mess...it because everyone is so stressed. No one is
born angry... yet people cannot see...that we all "inside" look
alike... yes you and me. In my disabled state...I am so so free.
I wear a "Superman mask" every day...because I have to save
you first...then me. Do not run away and hide because you
do not know me...sitting down for a spell...and talk...it for
free. You are "Paul Buyun" and I am "John Henry"...and we
play on the same team. Yet "freedom of speech" and "right to
assemble for all"...for many is it "just a dream". I know the
high and low from inequalities...because at 6'5" and black...
sometimes I stand in the back to reflect and see...all of whats
happening around me. And whether streetwise or talking like
a King...we ALL have lost our focus...for achieving the same
things. You see richer or poorer at the end of time...it will not
matter in heaven. For now we can all still "take a breath"...
while many cannot anymore because of..."their death". Add
to this laundry pile a pandemic...and another case of injus-
tice...captured for film for all to see. We top this all off with
"protect and serve"...but not everyone thinks its deserved.
While we ALL need this service of protection...its no fun to
do...because a few bad apples do not want to be outdone.
Now our "laundry bag" is full for all the world to see. Our
world is breaking up...it's "tired"..."frustrated" with a sense of
"hopelessness" leading the way. But what about all the good
things in life...being done today. Like a thoroughbred finishing

strong at the end of a race...we have to do the same and keep up the pace. Our "pile of dirty clothes" lay on this floor...a reflection on our "feelings"... oh a chore. What will this smell like tomorrow you may ask. But today the scent...is being "unmasked". Because "yours is mine"...we are the same...yet we cannot talk about our problems to each other... oh what a shame. Expressions of sympathy are being spoken...yet cannot be heard... over the loud roar of the looting taking place on the "same floor". So those who care like me and you...choose a simple act of kindness...while most have no clue. So picking up these clothes together is our start...or we can "choose to let them lay there for forever" on our hearts. Because there will always be clothes on this damn floor...but we can and must choose together..."to soar". Only one person I know who has seen this all before...its God now standing there knocking at our front door. So "our mission" is simple and plain as it can be..."Caring and Sharing" with each other is key. There is no difference between you and I...so just choose to give it a try. Sit with someone today not like "you"...if given the chance they will speak...and talk too. For now is a time for "unity and a focus"...to reach and teach each other together...so let us both start with today.

It Means Nothing Until It Happens To You

"He leads my "team of experts" so happy to see them shine."
- For my Neurosurgeon Dr. William Hicks and his staff

Physicians and their staff are people too...just like us all. Same feelings and problems but what is important to us at that time are only their "successes". You see when they are working with us...all that matters is their "title". With this on the table now let us get started. First whatever they brought into work that day "disappears from view" and is replaced with "caring for us". Whether direct or showing compassion is all the same...we just wanted to get better. There assemble "team" is an orchestra playing the "same tune" too. All playing their part in "our unique symphony" keep their timing with the Conductor. While we are thinking about relationships important to us they are too but with a twist. To them all...the most important relationship is with that patient and nothing else matters. You see our day could end very differently from where it started. With them trying to "defeat a foe" with their instruments fighting on our behalf. The key is them "listening to everything"...our heart beating in tune with all the sounds of surgery or procedure going on around them. Working with "strength of a Lion" but with the "dexterity" required to save our life. You see as we lay there vulnerable...they respect "us" and it shows. So always "think first" then ask a simple question to everyone you meet. These 3 words while small in stature carry a great meaning. So say them with pride by asking..."How Are You". They will appreciate it and so will you.

My Legacy

What do you want your legacy to be...a statement not a question. For me it is simple. Sharing myself with others. Then they share our conversation with others in their circle of friends. And before you know it...a legacy is born. Now my efforts to "impact 1 life" turns into infinitely more. I see my small effort grow into something larger than life itself. My efforts to come alongside that "1 person" have now expanded to many. Therefore "my legacy" is written for me. Helping people find out about themselves is my goal in life. Which leads them to ask others questions about life. Which leads to more and more questions. It is needed and wanted by everyone. But not for the "faint of heart" because it takes work. We are learning things together...about each other...life. And God is happy because we are learning together...and not alone.

THE 3 PEOPLE I KNOW...

There are 3 people inside of me. The "person you think I am". The person "I think I am". And then the "Real me". I have found the "REAL ME" which is flaws. But God has turned my "flaws-self" in his..."diamond" by trading out my old perceptions and self-centered attitudes for a new set attitudes that God has develops in me. Out of a renewal of our thinking comes change. Change in my speech pattern. Change in my perceptions about things. More important though... "Change in my behaviors". What I choose to think and dwell on now is still the same...but knowing "my mind" is the key. When you guard "your mind"....you "guard your peace". The "3 people in me" today are pulling and tugging all the time like a game of "tug of war" inside. But I only have to focus our the last one... the "real me". The one that helps others although I cannot do the things I used too. Using my Spiritual Gifts all I need these days though. It gives me the chance to recognize how that "picture of me" now is the true picture. And that God holds it and me each day in his hands. This verse resonates today for all if we choose to listen "carefully and closely". That means us both just focusing and receive comfort in these words...

> "You didn't choose me. I chose you. I appointed you to go and produce lasting fruit, so that the Father will give you whatever you ask for, using my name."
> —John 15:16 NLT

WHAT A WAY TO WAKE UP

"A good reputation is more valuable than costly perfume. And the day you die is better than the day you are born."
—Ecclesiastes 7:1 NLT

I know this one firsthand...this verse. The day of my Stroke something happened. I now know a valuable lesson. I was to meet a friend named Deborah Johnson. And when I did not show up...she automatically knew something was wrong. She told me later it was out of my "CHARACTER". You see if I said I was going to do something or be somewhere...well I did. Sometimes early because that was my "M.O." So she sounded the alarm to look for me. In the meantime I was on my apartment floor..."sleeping soundly". To be found many hours later...by another set of friends because they had heard the "alarm in her voice" to them. So they search for me too. Which is why they came looking for me in the apartment. So needless to say...that "my reputation" on that day saved my life. But that is not the end of the story... Because as I laid there "sleeping"...I went somewhere special. I saw something I never thought I would see..."God". And in that moment I was overwhelmed with a JOY and PEACE OF MIND never experienced before. But when he sent me back here...I knew that things would never be the same. Because on the glorious day..."I was re-born". Not to be "God" but to act like him with you and others I met. And share what he gives us every day..."LOVE".

KIND WORDS

"Kind words are like honey— sweet to the soul and healthy for the body."

—Proverbs 16:24 NLT

What happens to us when we are met with kind words from someone else. It makes us feel like we are on "Cloud 9". The minute they are expressed to us we get a "little pep in our step". Its makes us feel good. Sometimes it can make us feel proud of our accomplishment. Yet at times we cannot express these same feelings to others. Its because there is something happening in my own life that I am going to take out on someone else. This is why. There is something happening in my life. At the end of the day we reflect on others how we are feeling today. Yet it is not easily resolved by taking the high road and "singing the praises of someone else". But by doing so we put our total "focus" on them...and not ourselves. By doing this they get a compliment. We received the encouragement and support of God. It truly helps them and us.

LOVE YOUR ENEMY

"But I say, love your enemies! Pray for those who perse-
cute you! In that way, you will be acting as true children
of your Father in heaven. For he gives his sunlight to both
the evil and the good, and he sends rain on the just and
the unjust alike. If you love only those who love you, what
reward is there for that? Even corrupt tax collectors do
that much. If you are kind only to your friends, how are
you different from anyone else? Even pagans do that. But
you are to be perfect, even as your Father in heaven is
perfect."

—Matthew 5:44-48 NLT

Coming up to the holidays this passage was laid on my heart
today. Its about loving your enemies. Not some off the time
either. But all of the time. Do what...the people that don't
care for me. Love them. Why and how. Well it simple...I am
to give them the mercy and grace God has given me. I know
theres someone, somewhere that doesn't like me. Not for
anything more than they don't know my story. So in the same
instances Gods asking me to extend myself to those people I
may not care for. Oh its not that easy. But with his help and
guidance it can be done. Because we all need to be heard yet
to be heard we must listen. And this is where we go wrong at
times. Its not easy to do but try. It is a process for sure needed
in this life...by all of us. Because we are not going to be liked
by everyone we meet. I know I can be the light for someone
and "You can too".

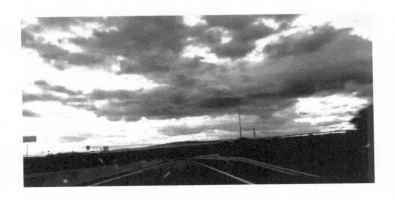

A View Inside..."My Near Death Experience"

"Sportspeople die twice in life...once when you lose your career then once at the actual end."

How has God been a refuge for you...is not a question asked but my statement. "He is in "me" because he saved me when he did NOT have too...is my reply. I know about all the "other things" of life because I chase them all the time. But never in "moderation". So in the end...I always had to search for more. Whether it was "my work" or "money" there was never enough of either one. But then "time stopped...dead in it tracks". And I did too..."dead in my tracks". But where I "stand now" is the blessing. Because he woke me up both physically and in spirit. Waking up from a "deep sleep of years gone by"...yet my memory when I woke up was not there. So waking up "this time" was different. You see all I have is "gratitude and joy in my heart" because of only one thing... the "Life" he gave me back. While I am the same man I was when I first fell asleep that day...I woke up with a different "mindset" now. Make your career and your purpose in life be the same. You will lose many careers for sure but "your purpose" in life is yours to decide. You see in the NFL as a player an abbreviation is what you are in that moment and it stand for..."Not For Long".

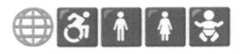

WE ARE ALL "ONE"

"FROM LISTENING COMES WISDOM AND FROM SPEAKING REPENTANCE."
—A CHINESE PROVERB

Below are people of all denominational but "of what". You see that up not to me to say. But I can see "myself" in..."them ALL". Because no one starts out knowing about "themselves" or "A God...". Its a real process for sure. With "on and off" times throughout our lives. Whether good or bad...no matter our culture or religion he loves us. So I shared an assignment for others to take. I ask them to "focus" and answer this question using "6 words". No less...more. Taking time to let it "marinate" on their "heart and mind". In this time of all this automation around us to use...I am a "relic". Back to a time when all we all needed and wanted was a...phone call. Reaching out and touching others. Letting each one "slow down their mind" as we chat about the "1 thing" that is important to them. Searching for our "North Star"...together. Because while there are many stars in the sky...what you are searching for its actually in your grasp. But it takes a partnership or two to navigate this thing called..."LIFE". So it is your choice to make each day..."We" or "Me". He still loved me even when I did not love "Me" as he does you. You see..."WE" all to share our failures and successes with someone else at some point.

My Question: "How does my Stroke help you in your life journey?"

"Life is better when done together!" - Deborah J. Columbus OH the person that sounded "the Alarm" when I did not show up a meeting that day.

"Faith Fear Few Frail Family Friend" - Reggie M. Columbus OH came to my apartment after Deborah sounded "the Alarm".

"Pray for health Take Prescribed medication" - Leon L. Columbus OH came to my apartment after Deborah sounded "the Alarm" with Reggie.

"Courage WALKING in absence of fear." - my WIFE Lisa S. Columbus OH

"Resilient teacher thought action and scripture" - Carson S. Son #1

"You can be resilient love wins" - Harry S. Son #2

"Slowed you down slowed me down!" - Pierce S. Son #3

"Once a man...twice a child..." -Edith "Mamae" D. West Point GA "My 2nd Mom and Cousin

"James shows God leads the way." - Loida L. East Hampton NY "My 3rd Mom" and Close Friend

Loida L. East Hampton NY "My 3rd Mom"

"Relentless, graceful, caring, faithful, loving listener" - Mark R. Kalamazoo MI and "My Best Man" in our Wedding

"Makes me think about Tough Challenges!!! 😊 👍" - Joe S. Columbus OH Father In-Law

"I appreciate good health, family, Grace." - Kathy T. Louisville KY and the Wife of my deceased brother Morris Thornton

"Continue to hone my professional skills." - Yvonne K. Columbus OH and Speech Therapist

"God makes no mistakes cherish life." - Larry D. New Rochelle NY and Cousin

"Your miracle reaffirms my faith everyday! 🙏" - Ray S. Middletown NY

"...quick to listen, slow to speak...". --- JAMES 1:19 naturally :) - John R. who baptized me at age 57 and a close friend Columbus OH

"YOUR STRENGTH AND TENACITY IMPRESSES ME" - Loxley "Animal" R. Birmingham England

"You've demonstrated Gods heart towards me." - Will D. Columbus OH

"Trust God. Let People help. Surrender." - Gabrielle T. Columbus OH

"Hopeful, Encouraged, Strong, Courageous, Dreamer, Purposeful" - Christian M. Columbus OH

"YOU are more DEPENDENT on CHRIST!" - Doug C. Scottsdale AZ

"TRUST, LOVE, HOPE, SERVE, INSPIRE, PERSEVERE!!!!" - Becky S. Columbus OH

"Love God With All Your Heart" - Renaldo "Skeets" N. Silver Spring MD

"With God All Things Are Possible" - Kevin H. Columbus OH

"You give me joy every day" - Jimmy H. Boise ID

"GOD always heals physically emotionally spiritually" - Robin D. Columbus OH

"The Lord has sent a witness." - Paul L. Boston MA

"Shit happens. Keep fighting. Never surrender." - Kyle A. Columbus OH

"It teaches me to slow down" - Sarah W. Columbus OH

"I see Jesus shinning through James" Jean Paul T. Columbus OH

"Grateful Thankful Special Appreciative Fortunate Blessed" - Cassandra S. Philadelphia PA

"You. Showed. Me. Anything. Is. Possible." - Jay R. Columbus OH

"Body is Weak...Soul Is Strong" - Antonio C. Seville Spain

"Step back. Look at Big Picture." - Joel P. Columbus OH

"Slow down, follow God's plan together" - Kadin L. Palma OH

"Clear thinking surrounded focus impressive future" - Arthur "AJ" A. Columbus OH

"To let go and let God love ♡" - Mark B. San Francisco CA

"1) Encouragement 2) Faithfulness
3) Hopefulness 4) keep- Going
5) Friendship 6) Looking (up)" - Craig S. Columbus OH

"Strength doesn't come from a muscle." - Christy K. Columbus OH

"Learn to appreciate life and health" - Dr. Neil F. Greenwich CT

"Your opening eyes and educating others" - Bob M. Columbus OH

"You are an inspiration to all" - Robert W. Manhattan NY

"LOVE like no one is watching" - Meghan P. Columbus OH

"F stands for FACE • A stands for ARMS• S stands for STABILITY • T stands for TALKING • E stands for EYES • R stands for REACT" - David D. Columbus OH

"You inspire me to love life" - Anthony "Tony" H. Columbus OH

"Major Things Happen In Minor Moments!" - Khadevis "KD" R. Columbus OH

"Let God shine through your frailties." - John S. Columbus OH

"*Have faith in God and believe*" - Nick A. Stamford CT

"Get busy living! Get busy dying!" - Kris H. Columbus OH

"More blessed than before the stroke" - Andy H. Columbus OH

"Every day brings a new opportunity." - Bob G. Los Angeles CA

"God's gotcha, just where he wantsya." - Bill M. Columbus OH

"It Demonstrates God Faith In Action" - Pamela F, London England

"Accepting lack of control is freeing" - Gabe G. Columbus OH

"Adversity brings you closer to God🙏" - Tim C. Columbus OH

"Never look down only look up" - Maxine B. Cleveland OH

"Always provides a beacon of hope" - Brian W. Columbus OH

"Life perspective and slowing to listen" - Matt D. Columbus OH

"Encouragement, more God focused daily living" - Rye D. Columbus OH

"Compassion appreciation humility friendship unconditional love" - Alec S. Sagoponack NY

"Your life inspires this insight today" - Mark D. Columbus OH

"Freedom shown through limits and constraints." - Steven "Knife" C. Columbus OH

"Pretty much broken only for minutes" - Tiffany B. Atlanta GA

"God is not done with me" - Steven S. Columbus OH

"Never take your health for Granted" - Mr. Z Columbus OH

"God's Faithfulness in times of trouble." - Don and Sandy G. Sonesta Key FL

"True Strength is born Through Adversity" - John C. Columbus OH

"No Limits with God, despite Limitations!" - Dan P. Chicago IL

"My grace is sufficient for you." - Paul B. Columbus OH

"He already working on a few!" - Rasome W. Columbus OH

"Helps me understand through another's eyes." - Carol H. Durham NC

"Perseverance Love Hope Grace Fellowship Brotherhood" - Paul F. Columbus OH

"Life is precious, love with expectation." - Damon M. Houston TX

"Work. The. Hand. You've. Been. Given." - Michael F. Columbus OH

"I witness the awesomeness of God." - Joe N. Stamford CT

"Perspective brings focused urgency to conquer" - "JD" B. Columbus OH

"You dedicated your life to God!" - Ovelle J. Columbus OH

"Grace, mercy, miracle, Inspiration, patience, surrender.. 🙏 🙏 " - Roy C. Brooklyn NY

"Let light shine out of darkness" - Scott W. Columbus OH

"Today is a present be grateful! ♡ " - Jasmine T. Los Angeles CA

"Your gratitude inspires others to love!" - Tom T. Columbus OH

" ◆ ◈ACTION◈ ◆ " - Fred O. Brooklyn NY

"Reinforced belief it's all God's plan" - Carol K. Columbus OH

"Growth through reflection and attentive listening" - Mike M. Sea Isle City NJ

"I see God's glory in you" - Ken T. Columbus OH

"Live every moment in the moment ...my 6 ☺" - Dwayne A Detroit MI

"Slow down to connect with God" - Jonathan M. Columbus OH

"God's mercy and Grace never fail." - Maliki W. Los Angeles CA

"Faith, Hope, Strength,
Beliefs, Perseverance & Love🕊" - Lindy R. Columbus OH

"Seek first the kingdom of God" - Randy Columbus OH

"It makes me appreciate every day" - John M. Columbus OH

"You are surrounded by blessings: people." Mark D. Columbus OH

IN THE GAME...

As long as you are learning...you are in the "Game" called life. You will get there "one step at a time". So remember this exercise when you are having "mental challenges" in your day. SLOW DOWN...you are trying to move too fast. So whatever it is...start with "small things" first turning into the "big things" we want. Those things we are striving to achieve but at times "biting off more than we can chew" which means we cannot digest it properly. So this exercise will help you until we meet again.

Count 1
Count 2
Count 3
Count 4
Count 5
Take a breath...

Count 1
Count 2
Count 3
Count 4
Count 5
Take a breath...

Count 1
Count 2
Count 3
Count 4
Count 5
Now take a deep breath...

Count 1
Count 2
Count 3
Count 4
Count 5
Take another deep breath...

Count 1
Count 2
Count 3
Count 4
Count 5
Take a deep breath again.

You need to remember this drill. People who climb Mount Everest have to do this exercise after a distance to climb on the mountain...to reach the top. This exercise is done between... each step. So think about it...that lot of breathing between those "small steps". But it allows them to focus and "stay alive" first and foremost. That is why I am asking YOU to do the same..."FOCUS". Then you can serve in your "PASSION 🎯" versus "Just a Job"...so keep it up as a "Thriver" now.

THANK YOU PAGE

"Because we cannot worry about what's not promise to us which is tomorrow."
Stroke of Genius

Before the eyes can see, they
must be incapable of tears.
Before the ear can hear, it must
have lost its sensitiveness. Before
the voice can speak in the
presence of the Masters, it must
have lost the power to wound.
Before the soul can stand in the
presence of the Masters, its feet
must be washed in the blood of
the heart.

MY FINAL WORD OF ENCOURAGEMENT

What I have learned through this "experience" is a loaded question for sure...but I will unpacked it carefully and slowly. Before my Stroke I use to depend on "my mind" each day. It was all I needed so I "assume". Whether "corrected or not" I had a 50/50 chance of being correct. My mind was everything to me...but I loved you with "conditions attached". Then God took that all away with my Stroke. I stand before you now because of "HIS LOVE FOR ME". To see me now...its looking a you in "my mirror". I understand now that God can do anything in life and in death. You see I was gone according to my Doctors. They had used everything in their arsenal. Yet in "my death"...God brought me back to life again but with a slight twist - on his terms now to "Share and Care" with others. So my "faith" is still a "work in progress" and will never end. But it is "unstoppable" now because it is all I have.

You see when you come back "from nothing in your mind" the choice is made for you. Just feeling something I cannot "see or touch" but you know it is there. When going through adversity how do you explain the truly "unexplainable". When "words and numbers and memories are gone"...I can only describe it as "Alzheimer in reverse". Yet I have learned like never before that..."Adversity Introduces A Man To Himself". I add "Again" at the end of this of this quote is from Albert Einstein who I am sure in his lifetime like us..."went through something" to reach this conclusion. In closing there is truly "nothing under the sun" that has not been said before. Yet we all have a "style and audience" if we do not select and just let God pick them for us. Then by showing through our actions versus "preaching to them" they will hear "our voice" when others with the same message failed. By sharing "a smile" with someone that does not look like us as individuals it brings all of "the pieces connected into play and the breaches close". That is a "LOVE that is unconditionally" and desired by all.

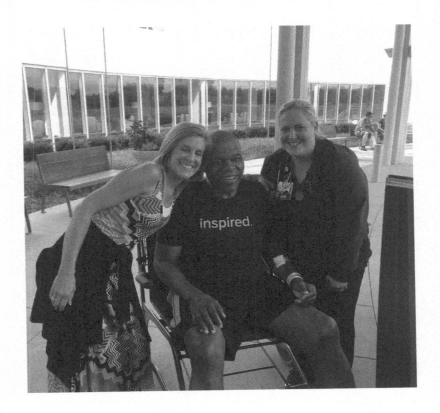

People "see my special needs" but I see us "all"... as special.
—James Thornton aka "Stroke of Genius"

You have in your hands a "Choice to Make" today. Definitely not tomorrow. You see in one fell swoop it can all be taken away..."your LIFE". Launching you into uncertain times and calamity if you let it. "Thriving" focuses on the beauty in life so I am going to show "you" what makes us right in life...is not our "religion".

ABOUT THE AUTHOR

James Thornton is a Stroke Survivor, Stroke Survivor Advocate, Mentor and now an Author. On June 5, 2018 he suffered a massive stroke. Found on his floor more than some 20 hours after, he was rushed to the hospital where the prognosis was grim. He was not expected to ever walk or talk or write again. It's called "Global Aphasia". So, writing for him truly is a gift from God. A former college football player who pursued a professional career, he became an executive with various firms, including the NFL, James is a "global citizen" who has lived and worked in over 15 countries. He was on the "go" all the time as an executive and as a speaker. He always had lots of questions about God and life, and then something happened which forced him to slow down - a Stroke. Even though his body was in great shape, his brain was not. This book is a collection of James' short writings telling of the "Journey" he is on now. Sharing his "struggles and success" in getting back all he can each day to encourage and inspire you. His inspiration is his wife and caregivers Lisa Showe. She has been there for him always and he loves her for this. Lisa and James live in Columbus, Ohio and have 3 sons Carson, Harry and Pierce with an extending family all over the world. This is written to Caregivers and Stroke Patients trying to best they can because everyone is a "Survivor" in life.

Made in USA - Kendallville, IN
45174_9781647469252
07.14.2022 1411